Bristol Medico-Historical Society

PROCEEDINGS

Volume Eight

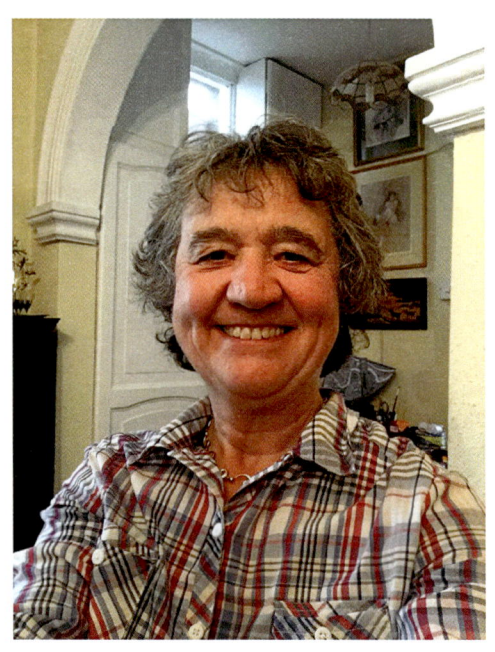

Lois M Tutton
EIGHTH PRESIDENT OF THE SOCIETY

Bristol Medico-Historical Society

PROCEEDINGS

Volume Eight

2016-2020

Edited by

Paul R Goddard

MMXX

Published by the **Bristol Medico-Historical Society**
Redland Green Farm
Redland
Bristol
BS6 7HF
© **Bristol Medico-Historical Society** 2020

First published in the UK 2020
Bristol Medico-Historical Society Proceedings Volume 8
ISBN 978-1-85-457100-7
Published by: Clinical Press Ltd for **Bristol Medico-Historical Society**

Redland Green Farm, Redland, Bristol, BS6 7HF, UK.

Contents

		Page
Frontispiece: Lois M. Tutton, President 2016-2020		2
From the president.....		7
A history of the management of Emphysema:	Nabil Jarad	9
Two madhouses of St Georges:	Peter Carpenter	55
Two medical chemists of Bristol:	Brian Vincent	63
A History of Caesarean Birth:	Tom F Baskett	76
Agatha Christie's use of poison in her novels	Janet Sellick	77
Dr Richard Smith	Mike Whitfield	89
Sir Francis Bacon	Peter Dunn	98
The Evolution of Pre-hospital Emergency Care	Tom F Baskett	98
The Hotwells Spa	Paul Main	99
All I want for Christmas is my two front teeth.	Lois Tutton	121
The History of MRI	Paul Goddard	130
The Poppy: panacea and plague	Gordon Stirrat	137
Swaddling: then and now	Peter Dunn	151
Scottish doctors at the Russian Imperial Court :Bruno Bubna-Kasteliz		167
Scottish doctors and the slave trade	Mike Davidson	176
Vesalius, the angry father of human anatomy :	Walford Gillison	184
Bath War Hospital (1916-1919)	Francis Duck	196
John Dunn and the Zulu War	Peter Dunn	224
Shaking Hands With the King of the Zulus	Paul Goddard	246
The history of the Victoria Cross	Chris Ackroyd	248
Eubulous Williams	Mike Whitfield	252
TB Meningitis	John Powell	262
In memorium		267
The scoiety's programme 2016-2020		268

From The President.....

What a four years! I have really enjoyed my term as President of the Bristol Medico-Historical Society (BMHS) from 2016 - 2020. This was nearly derailed for me with a surprise diagnosis of bowel cancer in December 2017 for which I underwent major surgery to remove a fist-sized tumour and a foot of bowel. The need to chair BMHS meetings and the support of all the members really helped me *'get up, get out of bed and put my troubles out of my head'* and recover. Thank you all for all your support and encouragement.

One of the major highlights of my term has been the British Society for the History of Medicine (BSHM) choosing Bristol for their biennial conference venue and the chance for our local society to help host a most successful event. M Shed was chosen as the conference venue due to its central location, facilities and views and it proved to be an excellent choice. With typical indomitable spirit a small committee of myself, Prof. Paul Goddard, Dr Peter Carpenter and Dr Michael Whitfield found places for evening events (a quiz at M Shed, a Fish and Chip supper while sailing on The Matthew round the harbour), tours to the John Wesley Chapel and New Room, Glenside Museum and the Jenner Museum and the conference dinner. We worked alongside a similarly dedicated team from BSHM and after numerous Skype meetings and occasional visits from BSHM committee members the event opened for over 125 delegates in the second week of September 2019 and the sun shone throughout! There were excellent talks packed with delegates running concurrently in three rooms throughout the three days of the meeting. The photograph on the following page was taken at the Conference Dinner which was held in the Sansovino Room of the Harbour Hotel on Corn Street (the old banking hall of Lloyds Bank).

Chris Derrett (president of the BSHM) greeted guests who included Lord Mayor Jos Clarke, her consort of the evening Stephen Williams, Prof. Steven West (Vice-Chancellor of the University of the West of England), Ros Kennedy (president of the Anchor Society) and our own Peter Carpenter (president of the Bristol Medico Chirurgical Society). Dr Jazz provided accompanying music .A memorable evening.

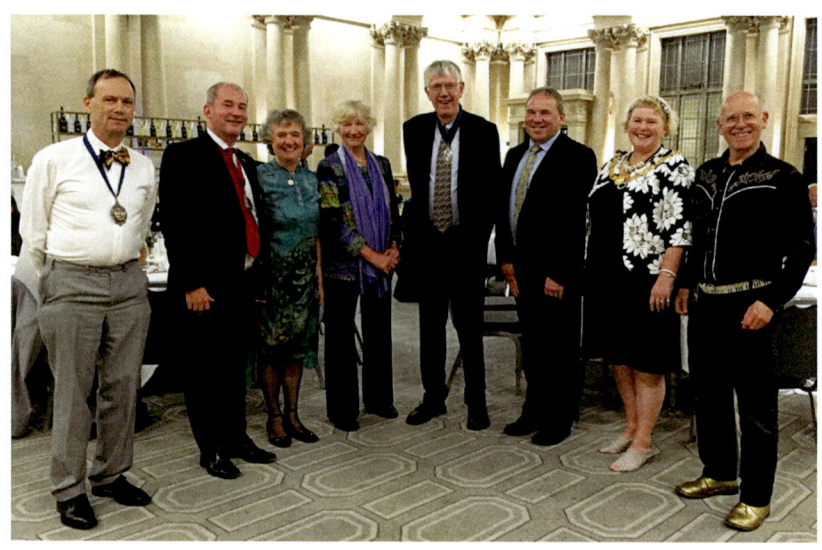

Presidents and guests at the BSHM meeting (September 2019)

We have been treated to some excellent talks at our local society meetings and I will let you read the following papers to remind yourselves of their content and a big thank you to all the contributors.

A big thank you also to Prof. Paul Goddard for his hard work collating the papers, typesetting them and supervising the printing of the proceedings. Dr Peter Carpenter has been as hard working as ever in his role as Honorary Secretary arranging meetings and the calendar of lectures while also being President of the Bristol Medico Chirugical Society in a very difficult year of Covid 19, lockdowns and all the ramifications preventing large groups of people physically meeting together since March 2020. The societies will find ways round this and it may mean a more digital approach for the time being but the research and recording of medical history is too important for it to stop and will prevail come what may.

Lois Mary Tutton MSc, BDS
President Bristol Medico-Historical Society 2016 - 2020

The History and Future Treatment of Emphysema
Emphysema Valves, Emphysema Coils and Volume Reduction Surgery

Dr Nabil Jarad PhD FRCP

Consultant Respiratory Physician
Bristol Royal Infirmary
Bristol BS2 8HW

E mail: Nabil.Jarad@uhbristol.nhs.uk, Nabil.Jarad@icloud.com

Presented at the Bristol Medico-Historical Society meeting on October19th 2016

Abstract

Emphysema is one component of the spectrum of Chronic Obstructive Pulmonary Disease (COPD) a condition that affects at least one million persons in the UK.

Emphysema is a lung tissue damage induced mainly by cigarette smoking. For that reason, the condition has been treated with nihilism by health care workers.

Breathlessness, weight loss and fatigue are the main manifestations. Up to recently only symptomatic treatment including inhaled bronchodilators, oxygen therapy, anxiolytic agents and opioids were provided to treat breathlessness.

However, over the past ten years, new interventional modalities of treatment have been introduced which revolutionised the outlook ofthis condition. This article looks back at the history of emphysema management and examines the exciting future of emphysema management.

The evening lecture on this subject was delivered by the author on Monday 19 October 2016 at the Create Centre – Bristol during the 2016 Annual General Meeting for the Bristol Medico-Historical Society.

Background

COPD is a progressive disease characterised by airflow obstruction. The obstruction is not fully reversible with current therapies. It is induced by cigarette smoking, exposure to other noxious gases including biomass fuel, and by age. Rare congenital causes such as alpha 1 anti-trypsin deficiency can cause emphysema at a young age. COPD affects the lungs mainly but other organs including the cardiovascular system, the skeletal muscles and the weight bearing bones are also affected (GOLD Initiative 2016).

Nearly one million patients are affected by COPD in the UK, with an estimated another further two million undiagnosed.

COPD has two components; airway narrowing due to increase mucous gland and respiratory muscle constrictions and a damage to the small airways and alveolar spaces (parenchyma). The parenchymal component of COPD is emphysema.

The current management of COPD consists of two strands, the first is to treat symptoms, improve breathlessness and health-related quality of life: this normally happens by using bronchodilators. The second treatment strategies aim at reducing exacerbations, reduce the decline in lung function tests and improve survival. This strategy consists of smoking cessation, inhaled long-acting bronchodilators and inhaled steroids ((GOLD Initiative 2016).

The difficulty with emphysema

Emphysema is defined as a destruction of lung tissue beyond respiratory bronchioles. Up to relatively recently, the gold standard method to make a diagnosis of emphysema has been considered to be a lung tissue biopsy. The histological appearance of emphysema is that of small airway destruction, widening of air-spaces and absence of alveolar tethering (figure 1).

The obvious difficulty in obtaining lung tissue sampling in vivo stood in the way of developing diagnostic and in evaluating therapeutic methods.

The advent of high resolution CT scan has revolutionised our understanding of emphysema. CT scan has been able to accurately identify patterns of distribution of emphysema as well as its extent. Recognising upper lobe predominant disease, lower lobe disease homogenous emphysema and patchy emphysema (figure 2)

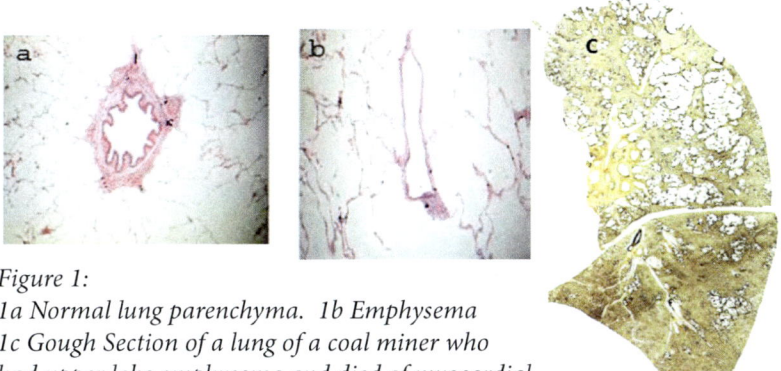

Figure 1:
1a Normal lung parenchyma. 1b Emphysema
1c Gough Section of a lung of a coal miner who had upper lobe emphysema and died of myocardial infarction.

enabled new thinking to develop methods to manage the disease interventionally. Most of the new work in describing the appearance of emphysema was made at the Bristol Royal Infirmary by Professor Paul Goddard (Goddard 1982).

The mechanism of emphysema is not totally clear. It probably results from lung damage by excess proteolytic enzymes in smokers. These enzymes come from the granules in neutrophils. In most people anti-proteases (anti-trypsin for example) are present in sufficient quantities to capture and neutralise the released proteases. Therefore, most smokers do not develop emphysema. When the anti-proteases

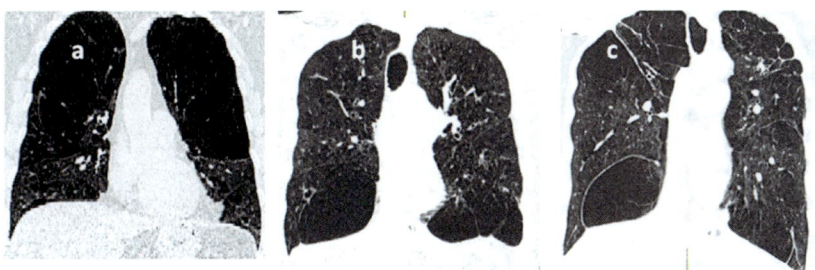

Figure 2: Coronal CT scan in 3 patients. –
Upper lobe emphysema (a),
lower lobe emphysema (b)
and patchy emphysema with bullous formation in the right lower lobe (c).

are insufficient in quantity or in quality, tissue damage is thought to result in emphysema (Abboud RT, et al).

Recently, studies from bronchial casts in explanted lungs showed that emphysema occurred early in disease progress (Hogg J ERS 2016) (figure 3). These studies also revealed that, contrary to previous assumptions, the process of COPD and emphysema starts from the periphery of the lungs and gradually extend centrally as the disease

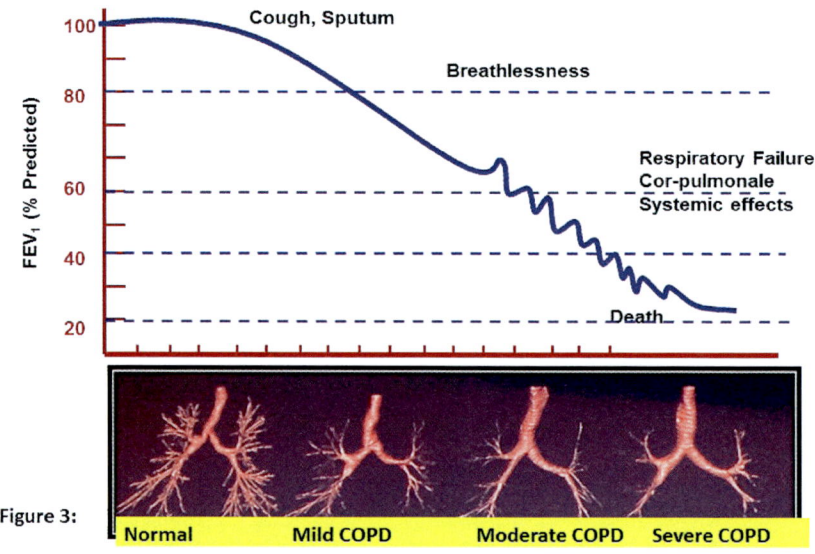

Figure 3:

Figure 3: Decline in lung function with age in smokers with emphysema. Below: bronchial tree casts of patients with different stages of COPD. Please note loss of peripheral and small airways even in the mild form of COPD. (Hogg J. European Respiratory Society (ERS) meeting – London 2016)

process progresses. This is supported by studies on high resolution CT scans of the thorax (figure 4).

As emphysema advances, two pathological phenomena occur. The first is that the small airways get fewer in number (Diaz A 2010) and thinner and therefore become easier to either collapse and/or kink during expiration. This would account for the sudden reduction of flow seen on the flow-volume loop (figure 5).

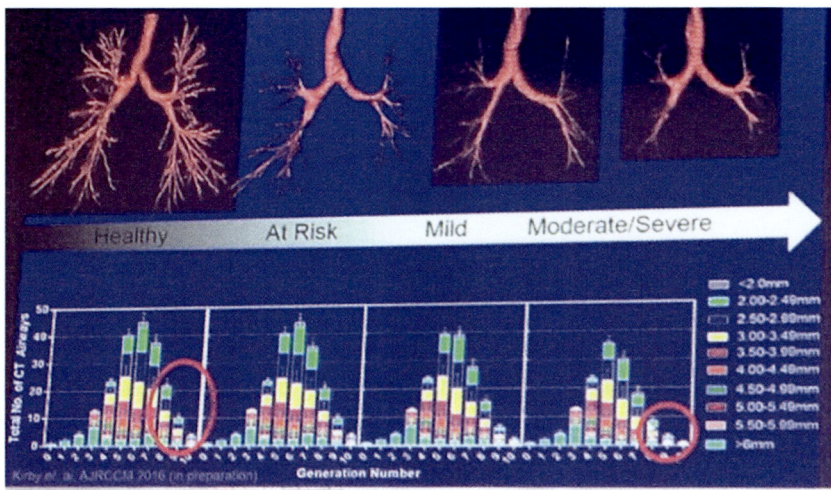

Figure 4: The bronchial casts of patients with emphysema – below this is a histogram showing the gradual loss of small airways on quantitative CT scans (red circles) Slide from Hogg J – ERS 2016

The second is a fusion of alveoli forming large spaces, in which the air does not get a gas exchange, thus forming air trapping (figure 6).

Air trapping or hyperinflation is responsible for the classic appearance of patients with emphysema. It is responsible for the pursed lip breathing, the increase in anterior-posterior diameter of the chest wall (kyphosis) and

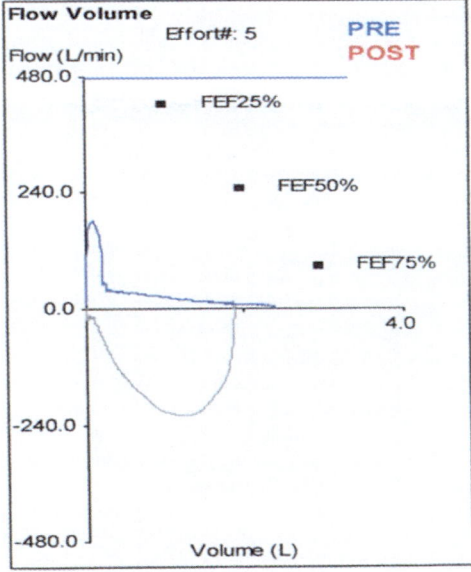

*Figure 5:
Typical flow-volume loop for emphysema. Note the sudden reduction of flow accounted for by collapse of moderate size and small airways at forced expiration.*

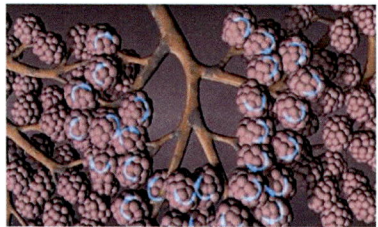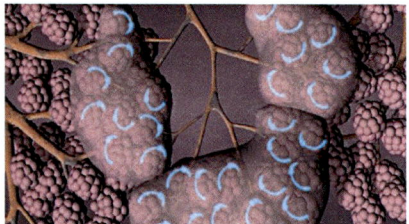

Figure 6: A schematic representation of (a) normal airways with intact number of small functioning airways and alveoli as well as good size airways and (b) emphysematous lung in which there is fusion of the alveoli causing air-trapping represented by the blue arrows and thinning of the airways. The thinning of the airways makes them prone to collapse during expiration.

probably in the failure to gain weight due to increase work of breathing in emphysema (figure 7).

The epidemiology of emphysema:

As the diagnosis of emphysema previously needed biopsy and autopsy, epidemiological calculation had not been possible. However, a recent study examined the degree of the presence of emphysema and the extent of emphysema on quantitative CT scan of the chest (Schroeder

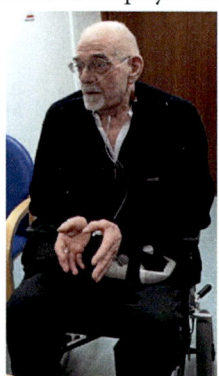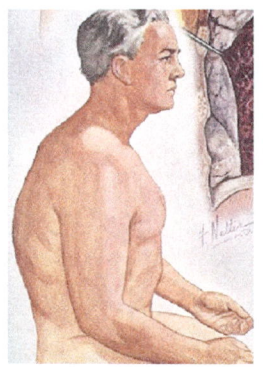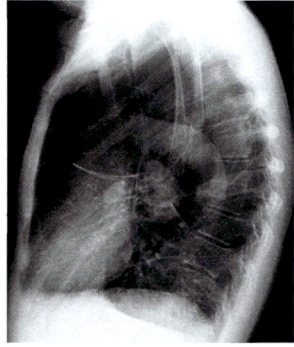

Figure 7: A patient with emphysema (a) – please note the reduced body mass index and the pursed lip breathing. (b) a schematic representation of the increase in anterior-posterior diameter (kyphosis) and (c) a lateral chest x ray of the patient confirming the kyphosis induced by lung hyper-inflation as well as low attenuation of the upper lung zones.

2013) in a large cohort of COPD patients enrolled in the COPD Gene Study. When examining the results of the study, emphysema, expressed as low attenuation area, was found to be highly prevalent when FEV1 reduced below 50% of predicted values and when FEV1/FVC ratio was below 50% (figures 8 a and 8 b).

The lack of available pharmacological treatment for emphysema has resulted in the development of non-pharmacological methods in managing emphysema. These are mainly interventional procedures.

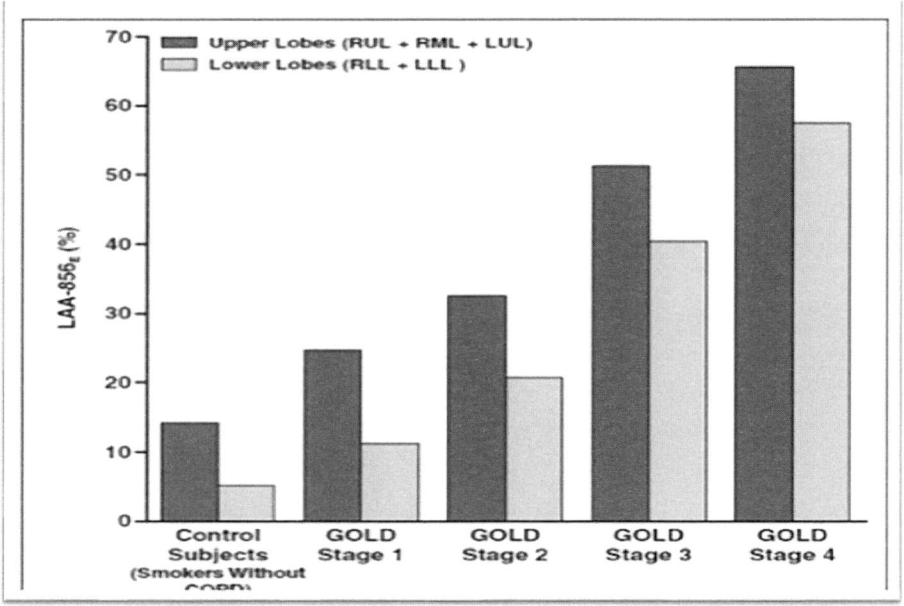

Figure 8a: Prevalence of emphysema expressed as Low Attenuation Area (LAA) on HRCT scans of patients with different GOLD stages depicting declining values of FEV1. Please note that when FEV1 declines below 60 % of predicted there more than 40% likelihood of patient having emphysema. From Schroeder 2013

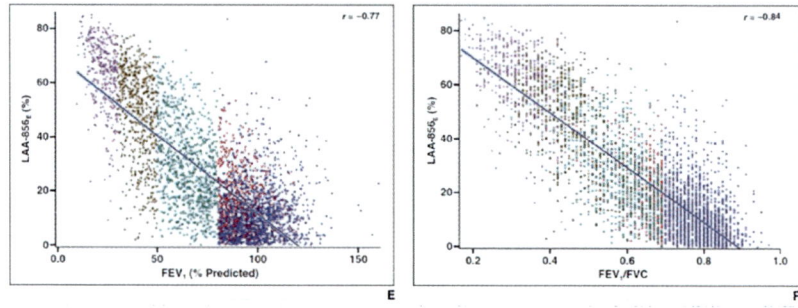

Figure 8b: The proportion of emphysema space on HRCT scan expressed as the Low Attenuation Area (LAA) Versus FEV1 (left) and the degree of Airflow obstruction expressed as FEV1/FVC ratio (right). This and figure 8a showed that not only the presence of emphysema but the extent of emphysema increases with reduced lung function (Schroeder 2013).

Interventional Management of emphysema:

Lung volume reduction surgery (LVRS):

In hyper-inflated lungs with severe air-trapping, removal of the most affected parts of the lungs was done on sound theoretical grounds. The intended benefits consisted of reducing dynamic hyper-inflation and restoration of the mechanics of the chest wall and the diaphragm which are compromised because of hyper-expanded lungs.

The first attempt to remove parts of the lungs in patients with severe emphysema was undertaken by Brantigan in 1950 who operated on two distinctive pathologies: removal of bullous disease and removal of diffuse emphysematous part of the lung. The procedure was done through thoracotomy.

In 1957, the results of 89 patients were available (Brantigan 1957). The study found clinical improvement in 75% of patients and in some it lasted for 5 years. The precise measurement of clinical improvement was not clear. No results in improvement in lung function tests were published. Mortality rate was 16%. Due to these shortcomings,

Lung Volume Reduction Surgery (LVRS) did not take off as a credible procedure until the 1990s.

In 1993 the concept and the procedure of LVRS was revived by Cooper and colleagues who evaluated bilateral LVRS in bullous disease. They found a maximum benefit from removal of large bullae occupying more than one third of the lung and with reduced FEV1 below 50% of their expected values (Cooper 1995).

In 1998, and despite some positive results, Healthcare Financing Administration (HFCA) halted the reimbursement of LVRS pending definitive evidence.

Several other studies reported advantages of LVRS. Criner (1999) reported improvement in lung function tests in LVRS for bullous emphysema compared to pulmonary rehabilitation. There was no difference in exercise capacity as assessed by the six-minute walk distance (6-MWD). Geddes 2000 on the other hand showed improvement in shuttle walk tests in LVRS of emphysema compared to best usual care.

High mortality rate from LVRS was reported in a study by Hillerdal in 2005 despite improvement in quality of life in those who survived the treatment.

The ultimate answer to the place of lung volume reduction surgery came from the National Emphysema Therapy Trial (NETT). NETT was planned as a prospective multicentre clinical trial comparing usual care in emphysema with volume reduction surgery. The recruitment period lasted from 1998 to 2002. A total of 1218 patients were included with 1:1 randomisation. The main outcome was exercise capacity using a maximum workload on cycle ergometer. Survival advantage was the second main outcome. The duration of follow-up was 5 years.

The study found that in all participants LVRS offered a small improvement in exercise capacity over medical treatment. There was no survival advantage over usual medical care. However, further sub-analysis demonstrated that patients with prior good exercise capacity and non-upper lobe emphysema did not have a functional gain and suffered highest mortality rate. This contrasts with patients

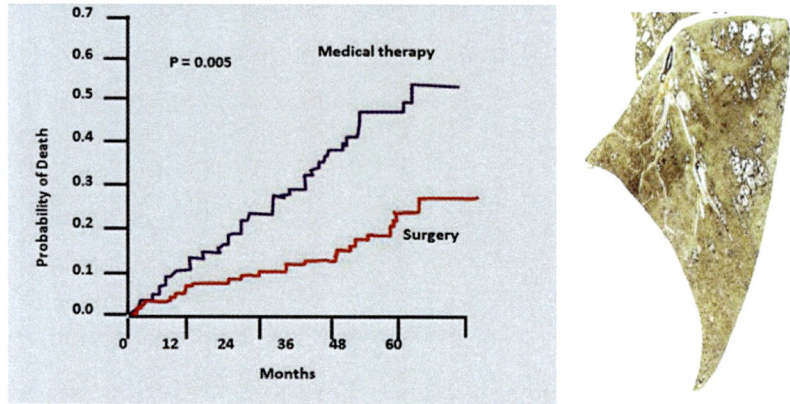

Figure 9: Favourable survival curve in surgically treated patients in a sub-group of patients in the NETT trial – those with upper lobe emphysema and poor exercise tolerance.

with upper lobe disease and poor exercise tolerance who gained the best survival advantage (figure 9).

The 30-day mortality rate in the LVRS group was tenfold greater than those in the medical group (2.2 and 0.2 respectively). The 90-day mortality rate in the surgical group was four times greater than in the medical group (5.2 and 1.2 respectively).

The morbidity rate of LVRS was also considerable leaving 28% of patients in nursing homes or being re-hospitalised within 30 days of the procedure. Despite all these, NETT has not increased enthusiasm in utilising LVRS as a method of treatment of emphysema.

Separately to NETT, centres with high volume of LVRS published more upbeat results compared to NETT. In a retrospective analysis by Weder et al (Weder 2009) found persistent improvement in efficacy of staged bilateral video-assisted thoracoscopy treatment in 225 patients with heterogeneous and homogeneous emphysema. Improvement of FEV1 and 6 MWD was seen in equal measures in the two study groups. The improvement lasted for 36 months. Lung transplant was obviated in 64% and 73% of homogeneous and heterogeneous emphysema respectively after 5 years of the study (figure 10). One-month mortality rate was 2.3% in both groups.

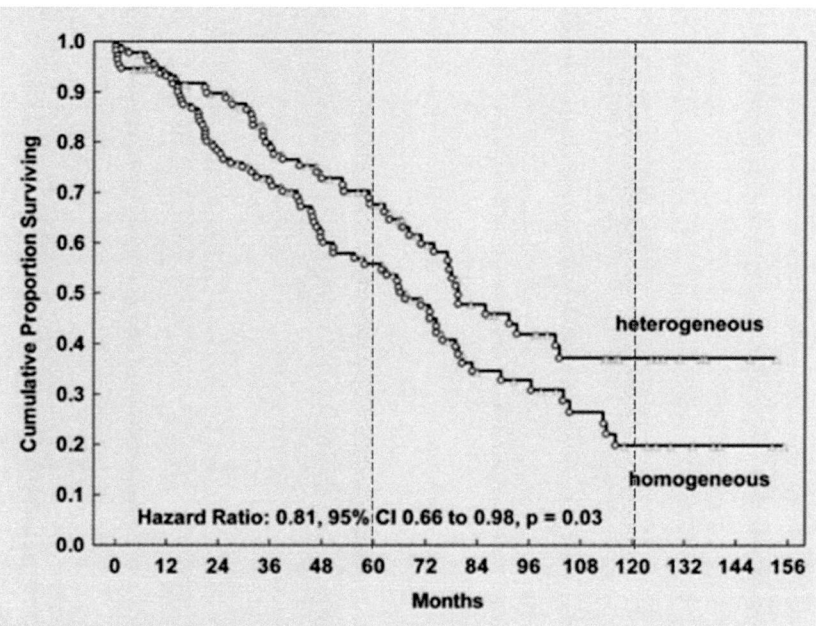

Figure 10: Favourable survival curve without transplant in surgically treated patients with heterogeneous and homogeneous emphysema. Weder (2009). Note the high survival rate at 5 and 10 years, in particular for patients with heterogeneous emphysema

Despite this study, LVRS remained an unattractive method of managing emphysema patients except in a small selected group. The popularity of LVRS remained low among thoracic surgeons as well as respiratory physicians (McNaulty 2014).

More recently, the role of LVRS has witnessed resurgence. This is mainly owed to the introduction of endo-bronchial volume reduction therapies. The introduction of the multi-disciplinary team meetings in which thoracic surgeons take part raised the interest in thoracic surgery as a method of LVRS and management of bullous disease. Many thoracic surgeons have taken a fresh look at the results of the NETT trial. This is owing to several reasons:

- Developments of new stapling methods with less possibility of air-leak.

- Reliance on differential perfusion scores between the target lobe and the adjacent lobe.
- Development of risk scores, with high risk includes composite factors: TLco < 20%, FEV1 <20%, pulmonary artery pressure of over 45 mm Hg, and co-morbid conditions.

For all these reasons, a prospective clinical trial (CELEB) is currently underway. The trial compares various subjective and objective outcome measures of LVRS versus endo-bronchial valves insertion in emphysema including lower lobe disease.

Endo-bronchial management of emphysema:

Endo-bronchial management of emphysema is a minimally invasive method of volume reduction. Several techniques have been developed and investigated over the past ten years. These methods are outlined below.

Tables 1a and 1b show broadly the criteria for referral and acceptance for volume reduction therapies.

Table 1: Criteria for referral (Table 1 a) and criteria for acceptance (Table 1b) for volume reduction therapies

(FEV_1) < 50% of expected values
Stopped smoking Undergone pulmonary rehabilitation programme
Modified MRC Breathlessness Score >2 COPD assessment Test score (CAT score) > 15
No major co-morbid conditions

Table 1 a

Has emphysema on chest CT scan
High air trapping – residual volume over 170% predicted
Rule out 'uncontrolled pulmonary hypertension' (degree depends on the proposed procedure valves, coils or surgery)
No major co-morbid conditions

Table 1 b

Endo-bronchial valves:

Endo-bronchial valves are one-way devices which, once in place, prevent air from entering while allowing the air out of the lobe. The aim is to collapse the target lobe and reduce its pathological influence on the better lobes in the lungs. The procedure effectively mimics LVRS but without removal part of the lungs. Unlike LVRS it is employed effectively in upper lobes and non-upper lobes.

Two valves are currently used- the zephyr valve (Pulmonx, Redwood City, California, USA) and the Spiration valve – Olympus Inc (figure 11).

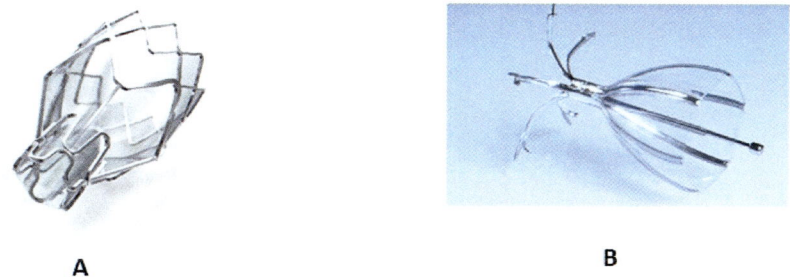

A   B

Figure 11:
The Zephyr valve (Pulmonx) (A) and the Spiration (Olympus) valve (B)

Most of the evidence has come from the Zephyr valves, although large studies are now either underway or have been published in abstract forms. The first generation of the zephyr endo-bronchial valves was the Emphasis valve – (Emphasis-Redwood City, California). The valve consisted of three parts – the duck bell valve, the retainer and the seal (figure 12).

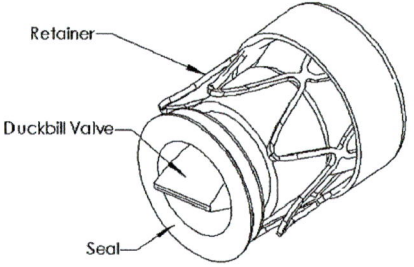 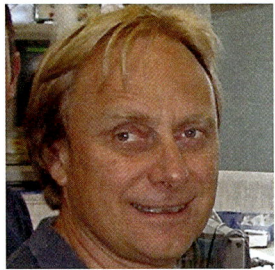

Figure 12: The emphasis valve (the first generation of zephyr valve). The valve consists of a retainer made of a nitinol cage, a seal made of silicon and the valve itself (duckbell) valve made of Silicon. The first animal and clinical work was published by Dr Gregory Snell (right) – (Snell 2003).

The valve was difficult to use and the procedure needed two operators, general anaesthesia, a rigid bronchoscope as well as a flexible bronchoscope. The work on these valves was first described by Snell and colleagues (Snell 2003). Their first step was to examine in vivo the efficacy of these valves on three sheep lungs aiming to familiarise themselves with valve insertion technique and with the post insertion effect. A post mortem removal of the lungs after valve insertion showed a collapse in the treated lobe in two out of three sheep. No intra-operative problems were encountered.

The valves were then inserted in ten patients with severe emphysema. The main aim of the pilot was to investigate safety and tolerability of the procedure. The average operative duration was two hours and forty-eight minutes. The procedure was found to be safe. No changes were seen in lung function or on CT scan in many patients. However, gas transfer (TLco) values had improved and lobar perfusion and ventilation diminished.

The introduction of the Zephyr (the author used this valve) (figure 13) and the Spiration valves (which the author has no experience in introducing) has simplified the intra-operative techniques. The procedure can be done by one or two persons under sedation through a fibreoptic bronchoscope (figure 14). The average time for valve insertion is thirty minutes although a pre-measurement of collateral ventilation using a follow catheter (see below) might take similar time.

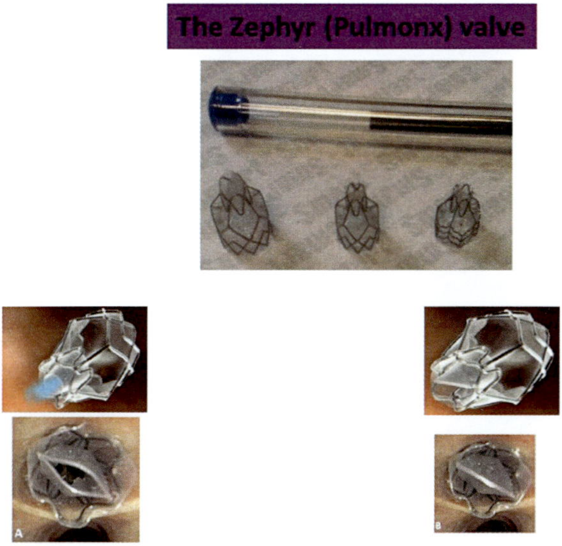

Figure 13: The 3 sizes of the Zephyr valve (above). The valves are the size of peanuts. The sizes are made to fit several sizes of bronchi. The valve opens during expiration (A) to allow air and secretion to leave the lobe and closes during inspiration (B).

The procedure is well tolerated and is reversible and valve removal is relatively simple in cases of complications or misplacement (figure 15).

A good outcome of endo-bronchial valve insertion hinges on the resultant lobe occlusion and subsequent partial or total collapse. When this happened, studies demonstrated significant improvement in various subjective and objective outcome measures including survival.

The procedure is illustrated in figure 14. A successful effect is illustrated in figure 16.

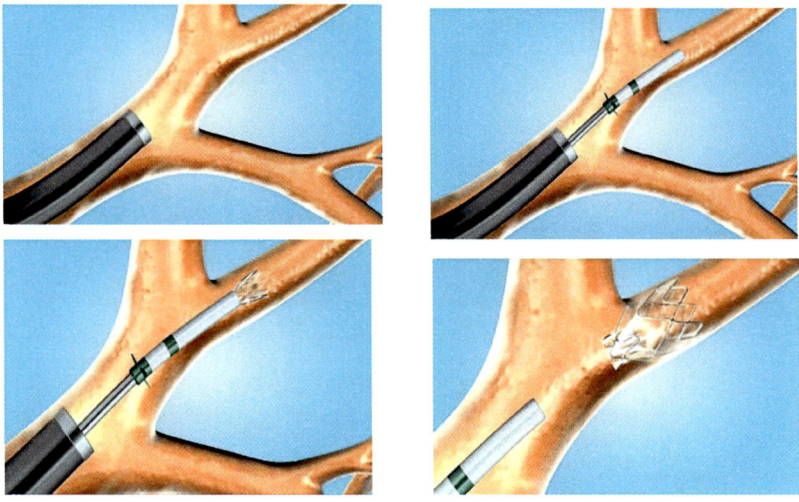

Figure 14: Image capture of insertion of an endo-bronchial valve in the apical segment of the left upper lobe.

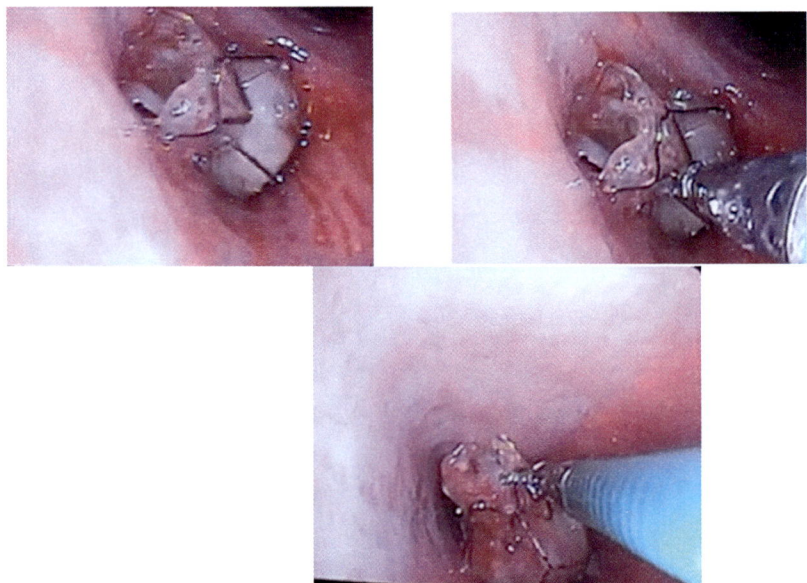

Figure 15: Removal of a misplaced endo-bronchial valve.

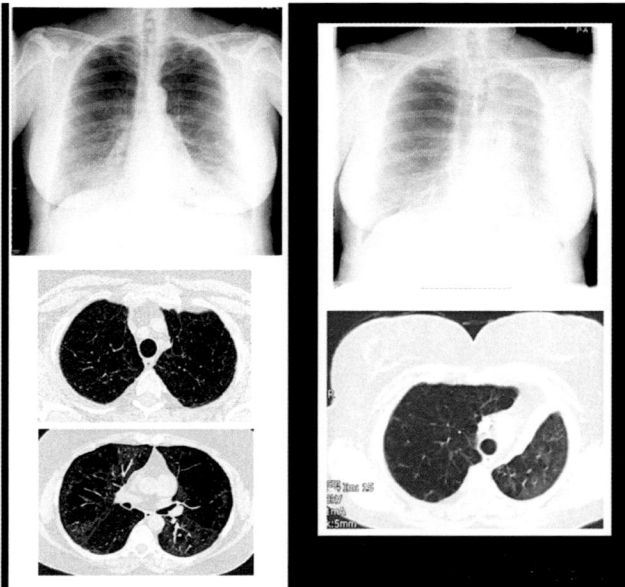

Figure 16:

The left panel shows a chest X ray and two CT slices before insertion and the right panel is of an X ray and a CT scan after insertion of endo-bronchial valves in a 71 year old lady.

The effectiveness of the Zephyr valves was sought in a large prospective clinical trial (the VENT study Scuirba 2011). This was a six months follow-up study conducted in the USA (321 patients) and in Europe (171 patients). The study was a 2:1 randomised study comparing valve insertion to usual care. The study was not blinded. The ultimate purpose of the study was to gain the approval of the US Food and Drug Administration (FDA) so that the practice may be rolled out in the US. The US arm and the European arm were reported separately.

The US arm of the study yielded disappointing results. Only a modest in-between group improvement in FEV1 of 6.8% was achieved. The improvement in 6-minute walk distance (6-MWD) was smaller at 5.8% in the group receiving EBV compared to the control group. The changes in FEV1 and 6-MWD were well-below the minimal clinically improvement difference (MCID). However, two subgroup analyses were undertaken to try and identify the best responders. The study found that high emphysema heterogeneity between the target and the adjacent lobes (in the US but not in the European study) and the degree of completeness of the inter-lobar fissure (in both studies) has resulted in a more favourable and meaningful improvement in FEV1, and

St George's Respiratory Questionnaire score (SGRQ) in the group who underwent endo-bronchial valve insertion compared to the control group (figure 17).

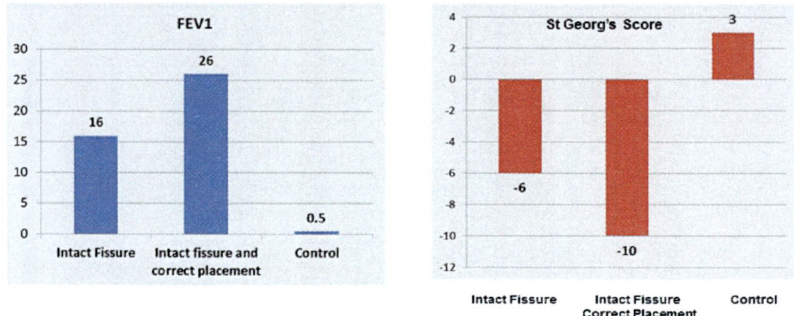

Figure 17: The results of the European Cohort of the VENT study. Please note a significant and meaningful improvement in FEV1 and SGRQ after insertion valves when the inter-lobar fissure is intact and after correct insertion resulting in lobe atelectasis. (Herth 2012)

As a result, selection of best responders from EBV has undergone a significant change. To put it simply, the likelihood of success and the benefit from the treatment are greater in the absence of collateral ventilation and with the correct placement of endo-bronchial valves. The selection for volume reduction therapies needs a minimum set of investigations. These are:

- high resolution computed tomography (HRCT) of the thorax,
- detailed lung function tests which include spirometry, lung volume measurement and measurement of gas transfer values,
- echocardiogram,
- 6-minute walk distance (6MWD)
- assessment of quality of life by either St George's questionnaire or COPD assessment test (CAT) score.

The role of lung isotope scanning by ventilation or perfusion is currently debatable but in the author's institute, a Single Photon

Emission Computed Tomography (SPECT) CT scan is obtained in almost all patients (figure 18).

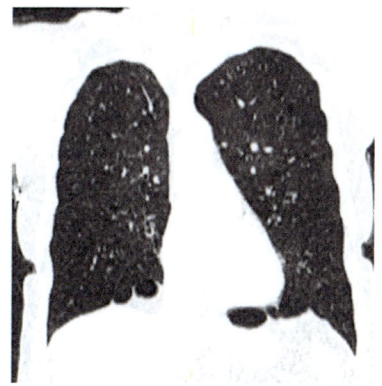 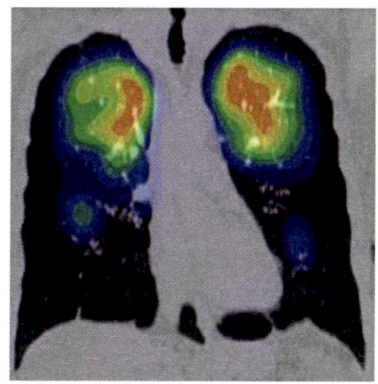

Figure 18: A single photon emission computed tomography (SPECT) in a 61 year old patient with lower lobe emphysema and heterozygote alpha1 anti-trypsin deficiency. Note that the CT scan (left) under-estimates the differential uptake illustrated on the SPECT scan.

Intact inter-lobar fissures:

The intactness of inter-lobar fissure can be assessed on 3D HRCT scans. Eyeballing the fissure has, until recently, been the standard method. Studies showed that eye-balling of the fissure had a good inter-observer agreement at a high degree (over 80%) and at low degree (below 60%) of fissure intactness. Greater differences between assessors was observed, however, when the intactness of the fissure ranged between 60-80% (Koenigham-Santos 2012).

Patients with intact fissures who were treated in the VENT study (Scuirba 2010) in both arms achieved good improvement in FEV1, SGRQ and 6 MWD. A retrospective analysis has shown, that in this group, a continuous improvement in FEV1 and significantly high survival after five years of valve insertion.

The degree of fissure intactness necessary to achieve post valve atelectasis has also been investigated. de Oliviera (2016) found that 75% or over was associated with atelectasis in 12/14 (85%). In contrast, fissure completeness of < 75% was associated with atelectasis in 1/9 (11%) of patients. Similar predictive values were reported in a study by Schumann et al (2015).

However, the use of fissure completeness alone by visualising the CT scan proved to show sub-optimal response in a single centre prospective sham blinded valve-sham controlled study (Davey 2015). In this study, a modest albeit significant response to valve insertion was achieved after three months of insertion of valve compared with the sham control arm. Chartis was assessed but not used in the entry criteria. None of the four patients who were later found to have a collateral ventilation (CV) positive pattern experienced lung atelectasis of showed increase in FEV1 following valve insertion. However, the procedure in this study had a low atelectasis rate with only 50% of treated patients achieving complete atelectasis.

The use of both; fissure intactness and Chartis catheter as methods to rule out collateral ventilations was associated with impressive results in another single centre open label study (Klooster 2015). Using both methods have been the policy in the author's unit from the outset of setting up this service.

More recently, automated methods of calculating fissure intactness have been developed and evaluated. The Stratx software (Pulmonx) is one example (figure 19).

Using this software, HRCT scans of previous clinical trials were analysed (Koster 2016). The degree of post-procedure atelectasis was taken as the main arbiter of the parameters obtained by this software. The study found that over 95% fissure completeness predicts therapeutic success in 82% of cases. This would suggest that valves could be inserted based on high fissure completeness seen on QCT scans alone with no need to using Chartis catheter.

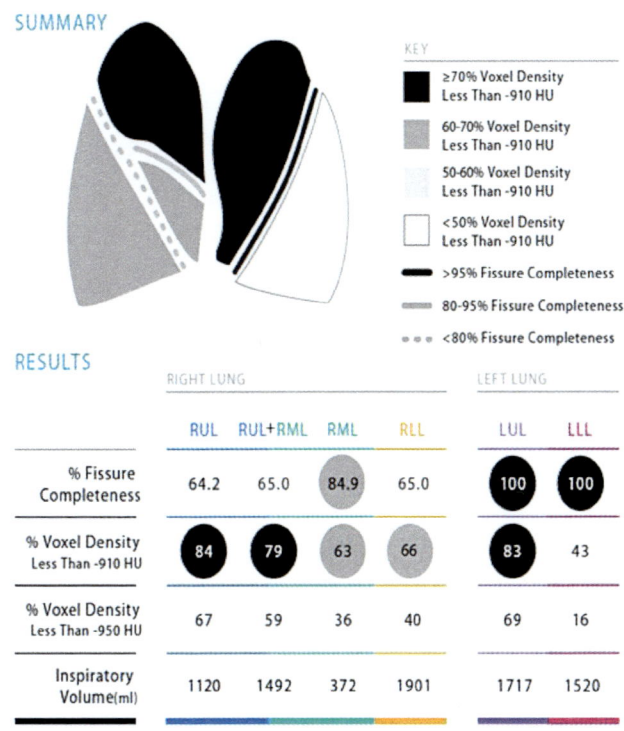

Figure 19: A quantitative CT scan using StratX software. The patient has highly heterogeneous emphysema and fissure completeness on the left side. A high degree of emphysema is observed in the right upper lobe (84% of the lobe) and in the left upper lobe (83%). The lowest degree of destruction is seen in the left lower lobe (43%). The left oblique fissure is 100% intact. - the right oblique fissure is 66% intact. This patient is likely to respond insertion of endo-bronchial valves in the left upper lobe without the need to use Chartis flow catheter measurement.

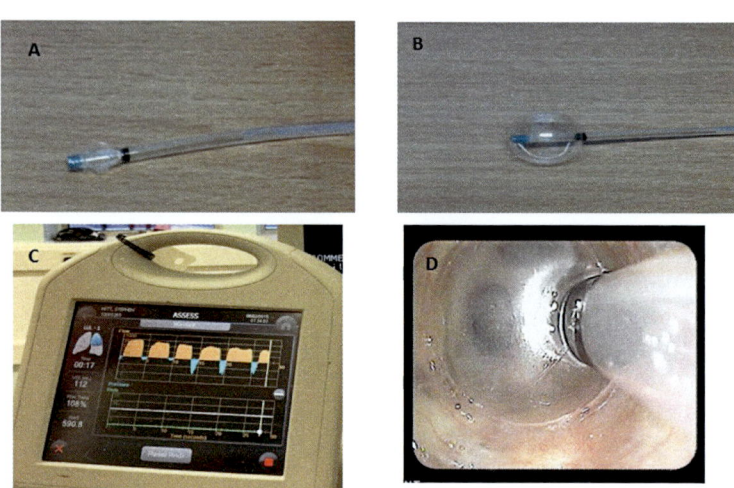

Figure 20: The Chartis catheter deflated (A) and inflated (B), the Chartis console [c] and the Balloon catheter inflated in the left upper lobe.

Figure 21: Three Chartis graphs from 3 patients. A: collateral ventilation (CV) negative pattern. Please note the decline in flow (orange) with time. The blue graphs help to identify a proper sealing of the catheter. CV negative pattern predicts post-valve atelectasis. B: this is a CV positive pattern which predicts no response to valve insertion. Pattern C: is a no flow pattern in a highly destructed lobe and bullous formation.

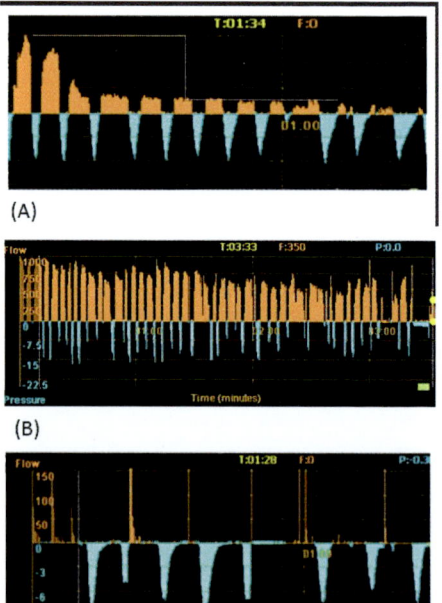

Assessment of collateral ventilation using endo-bronchial flow catheter (ChartisR):

The ChartisR system [Pulmonx – Redwood City- California USA) consists of a balloon catheter attached to a sensor based in a console (figure 20). The catheter is inserted through the working channel of the bronchoscope and inflated to occlude the orifice of the target lobe. A standard Chartis graph contains information displayed as a time- flow graph. Patterns of Chartis graphs are illustrated in figure 21.

A collateral ventilation (CV) negative graph shows typically a gradual reduction in the flow to the point of becoming invisible after few minutes of lobe occlusion. CV negative pattern would be an indication of high success rate after proper valve insertion. A CV positive pattern would show no reduction in flow over time after occluding the main bronchus of the target lobe. Valves inserted in patients with this type resulted in a high degree of failure. Other patterns of Chartis graphs have been described: the sudden loss of flow, the low amplitude pattern and the no-flow graph. Examples of each of these graphs are seen in figure 21. The sudden loss of flow is attributed to collapse in the airways and alveoli. The no-flow pattern is often seen in lobes with a large degree of destruction or in bullous disease. It has been suggested that, if either of these patterns are seen, relying on the fissure completeness on the HRCT appearance would be the way to decide to insert the valves or not. The low plateau flow pattern is thought to be a marker of small collateral ventilation with valve insertion likely to be unsuccessful.

The usefulness of the Chartis was reported in a study by Herth and colleagues (Herth 2013). In this study, a 350 ml volume reduction was regarded the clinically important volume loss after valve insertion. The study found that volume reduction occurred in most patients in whom the Chartis recordings showed CV negative pattern. In contrast, when the pattern was shown to be CV positive post valve volume reduction occurred in the minority of patients (figure 22).

The likelihood of lobes being CV negative, and therefore predicting a good response to valve insertion, varies between the different lung lobes. The likelihood of a CV negative pattern has been seen more

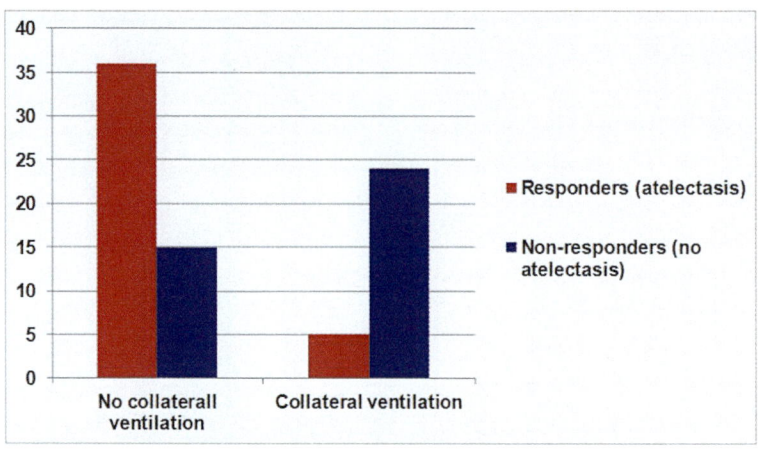

Figure 22: Rate of response according to the flow pattern- Herth 2013.

frequently in the left upper lobe and the left lower lobe, followed by the right middle lobe. The least likely lobe to show CV negative pattern is the right upper lobe. The fissures between right middle lobe and right upper lobes are often breached and the CV pattern in the right middle lobe is highly likely to be the CV positive pattern (Herzog 2016).

Evidence for Spiration Intra-bronchial valves (figure 23):

The Spiration Intra Bronchial valve (IBV) (Olympus) is an umbrella like valve. The valve is inserted via a fibre optic bronchoscope. Three sizes of the valve are used. Lack of collateral ventilation relies on evidence from HRCT.

Two prospective studies comparing valve insertion with standard care are ongoing. The SVS Reach trial aimed at recruiting 100 patients in a single centre in China with 2:1 randomisation with usual care. Change in FEV1 at 6 months point is the main point of the study. The study was reported in an abstract to the proceedings of the European Respiratory Society Conference in London – September 2016 (Shiyue Li – 5 September 2016).

The study found significant and consistent improvement in FEV1, 6-MWD, Breathlessness score at the mMRC questionnaire and improvement in quality of life as assessed by SGRQ and the COPD

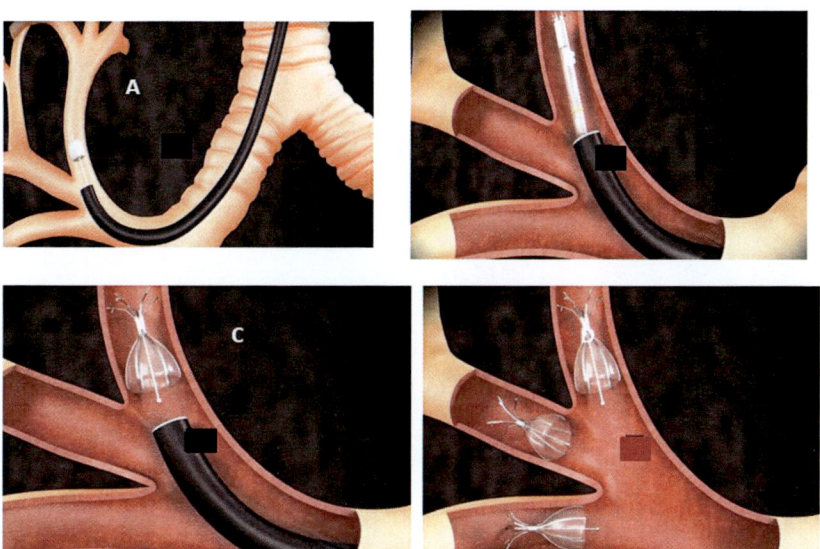

Figure 23: Insertion of Spiration valve. A. A balloon catheter measures the diameter of the airway. B. The valves deployed into the target bronchus and C: it is secure in place by . The stent mechanism and by 5 anchors. All bronchi leading to the target lobe are occluded (D).

assessment test (CAT) score. A larger multicentre study (EMPROVE) with similar design to the SVS study is currently recruiting in the US and Canada. The study is ambitiously aims at recruiting 270 patients in 37 centres.

Complications of endo-bronchial valves (EBV) insertion:

Several side effects and complications are expected after insertion of EBV.

- Infections and COPD exacerbations: Temporary increase in COPD exacerbation has been reported in up to 20% of the cases. These may represent true exacerbations or a reaction to the insertion of foreign body. Prevention of exacerbations is attempted by prescribing prednisolone and/or antibiotics prior to and after the procedure. However, there are no studies to support this practice.

- Chronic cough. This is a symptom that occurs in approximately 15% of patients. This is probably due to reaction to the presence of

- the valves in the bronchi. In the author's unit, cough necessitated removal of the valves in 2/88 patients.

- Pneumonia distal to the valve is seen in 3.2% of patients (figure 24). This should be managed in the usual way. Occasionally abscess formation in the emphysema spaces is seen.

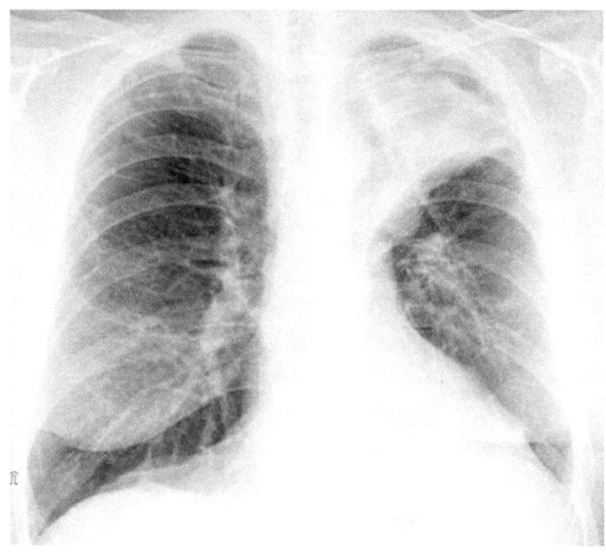

Figure 24: Pneumonic illness in the left upper lobe two months after insertion of endo-bronchial valves in the left upper lobe.

- Temporary haemoptysis is also encountered and often does not require any treatment. In the authors unit, anti-coagulation and clopidogril (but not aspirin) are withheld 7-10 day prior to valve insertion and re-started 72 hours after the procedure.

- Pneumothorax (figure 25) is one of the most serious complications of EBV insertion. The mechanism is thought to be a rapid expansion of the lobe adjacent to the target lobe after the collapse of the treated lobe. In some patients, adhesions were observed on video assisted thoracoscopy between the visceral and parietal pleura. Tearing of these adhesions upon expansion of the lobe has also been proposed as a mechanism of pneumothorax.

Pneumothorax happens in approximately 20-25% of patients. It almost always occurs in patients with complete fissure and a successful collapse of the target lobe. Over 90% of pneumothoraces occur within

72 hours. In the author centre all pneumothoraces occurred within a few hours from valve insertion. For that reason hospitalisation for 3-5 days and a daily chest X ray after valve insertion is recommended. A retrospective observation by Gompelmann and colleagues (2014) found that pneumothorax predicts a favourable late response to valve insertion.

The management of pneumothorax depends on its size, its clinical impact and the presence of broncho-pleural fistula. Observation is sufficient for patient with a stable small pneumothorax with little symptoms and normal oxygenation.

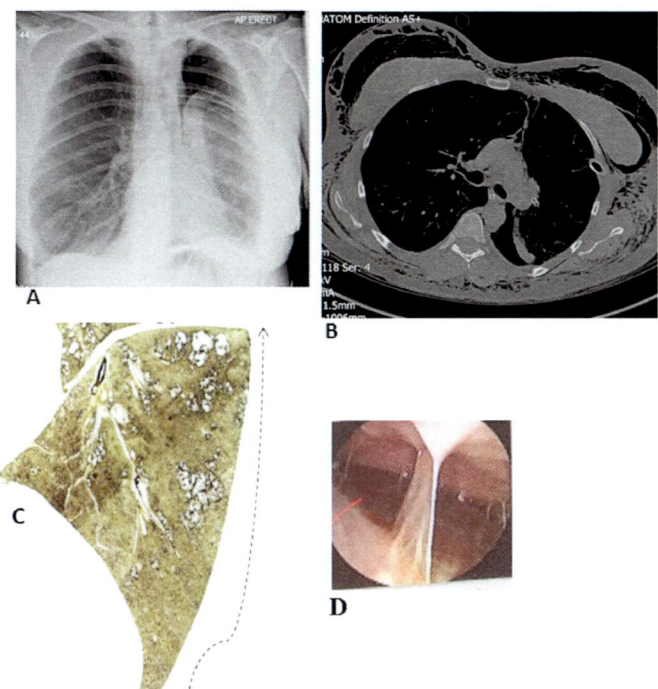

Figure 25: Pneumothorax after insertion of endo-bronchial valve in the left upper lobe. A. A chest X ray showing a pneumothorax in the left upper zone not responding to an inter-costal drain. B. A CT scan of the same patients 48 hour after showing Sub-cutaneous emphysema (the valves are in situ). C. A schematic representation of the mechanism of pneumothorax as a marker of expansion injury D: Adhesion between the visceral and parietal pleura which is probably another mechanism of pneumothorax.

A chest drain is inserted when the pneumothorax is severe or persistent. Less frequently, broncho-pleural fistula with continuous large leak may occur. In this group, surgical management of pneumothorax may be indicated. Removal of one or all valves may be necessary to stop pneumothorax in some patients.

Reinsertion of endo-bronchial valves after pneumothorax is possible and does not necessarily result in recurring pneumothorax. Some physicians however chose not to re-insert valves especially when the initial pneumothorax is severe.

Prevention of post-valve pneumothorax has been attempted by changing style of activities after valve insertion. One study demonstrated that avoiding cough by providing cough linctuses and reducing physical activities for few days has resulted in reduction in the rate of pneumothorax. The rate of thrombo-embolic events did not increase (Huebner 2015).

- Valve migration and dislodgement: Valves could be displaced after insertion leaving a gap and air leak that obviates the desired collapse of the target lobe. In the minority of patients the valves is dislodged and coughed up (figure 26). The reason for that is thought to be either incorrect insertion of the valves or choosing a smaller size valve. The latter can easily occur because bronchial oedema occurs during the Chartis procedure or during bronchoscopy. Oedema can reduce the calibre of the airways when measured. This may result in choosing a smaller valve size although in some patients, valve migration can occur for no obvious reason. Migrated and dislodged valves can be removed, and new valves are inserted. The procedure is technically easy and can result in good response.

- Formation of granulation tissue: Valves are foreign partly metallic bodies. Formation of benign granulation in the bronchial mucosa is common although the exact rate is not clear. Granulation is observed during bronchoscopy. Granulation tissue may be responsible for haemoptysis or loss of efficacy of inserted valves by changing the architecture of the bronchi (Figure 26). Valve removal and re-insertion after a few weeks can restore the function of the valves.

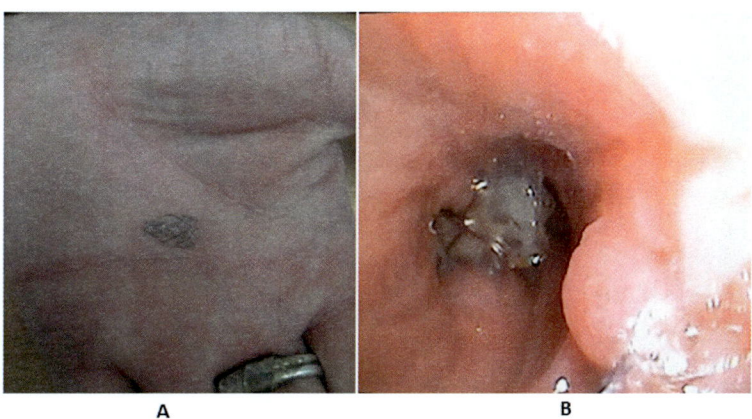

Figure 26: (A) Expectoration of a valve in a 54 year old patient. (B) Valve incompetence due to formation of granulation tissue in a 71 year old patient.

- Death can occur after endo-bronchial valves in up to 3%. Patients needing endo-bronchial valves are challenging. They have severe emphysema and often have other co-morbid conditions including cardiac disease induced by previous cigarette smoking and other co-morbid conditions. Despite a good selection process that considers clinical status as well as co-morbid conditions, death occurs at a rate of 2.5 % in the author's unit. The causes of death are ventilatory failure, pneumothorax, pneumonia, systemic sepsis, or massive haemoptysis. Careful observation and working closely with an intensive care unit would probably reduce but will not totally obviate death.

- Failure to respond. Failure of atelectasis after endo-bronchial valves occurs in 20-40% of cases. Most causes are speculative. This would include a) an under-estimate of fissure integrity, b) opening of collateral channels due to increase pressure c) fault in valve insertion d) migration or displacement of valve (sudden loss of efficacy) and e) opening of accessory bronchi. In all patients where loss of efficacy or failure to respond to valve insertion occur, a combination of CT scan and a bronchoscopy are advised. The reason is to look into wrong placement, peri-valve leak or missing bronchi that needed occlusion.

Evidence of increasing efficacy of EBV insertion:

The effectiveness of the valves has improved with improved selection process. As stated previously, the initial VENT trial found a small improvement in FEV1 and in exercise tolerance in all patients compared with the control arm. The outcome improved in sub-group of patients with highly heterogeneous disease and fissure integrity (Scuirba 2010).

A further sub-analysis of the European patients of the VENT trial found marked improvement in FEV1 and quality of life as assessed by St George's Respiratory Questionnaire when EBV was placed in patients where there is fissure completeness between the target and the adjacent lobes. Further improvement was found when there were signs of lobe exclusion (collapse) after valve insertion (Herth 2012).

More recently, the results of two prospective clinical trials are presented and are available on abstracts only. The first study was the first double blind sham controlled trial comparing endo-bronchial valve insertion with a sham procedure (Davey 2015). The sham arm consisted of bronchoscopy and Chartis balloon assessment. Of note, the selection criteria were based on fissure integrity only. Although Chartis assessment was made, this did not influence the selection of patients. The primary outcome was change in FEV1.

A total of twenty-five patients of each arm were recruited. At three months, the between group difference for FEV1 was 20.9 % (95% confidence interval of 4.3 – 37.5). There was a decrease of 400 ml for residual volume (RV) and 5.06 points reductions in SGRQ and 33 m increase in the 6 minute walk distance. The rate of volume reduction in this study was approximately 50%.

In another study, sixty-eight patients were randomised 1:1 for endo-bronchial valves and usual care. Patients were randomised only when favourable data from both Chartis and fissure completeness rate on CT scan. The six months results were impressive (Klooster 2015).

Compared to the control group, there was a marked difference in the number of patients achieving minimally important difference in all parameters in the valve treated group compared to the control group. The results included improvement in objective measurements

(FEV1 and residual volume), and in subjective markers (St George's Respiratory Questionnaire (SGRQ) and 6 minute walk distance. No placebo arm was used in this study.

A recent analysis showed that the efficacy of valve insertion as judged by subjective and objective parameters continued after one year although with some reduction in the magnitude for all parameters (Klooster 2016).

At the time of writing this article (November 2016), the results of the largest prospective trial (the LIBERATE trial) has not been published. LIBERATE trial is a prospective randomised control trial with 2:1 (valves: control) randomisation. The trial recruited 187 patients and has been run in over 50 centres in the US, two centres in the UK and one centre in the Netherlands. Patients included were those of high heterogeneous emphysema, over 80% fissure intactness and a CV negative pattern on Chartis tracing.

The study has two-phase follow up: 12 months after which a cross over phase start and 5 years follow-up for long term efficacy including mortality rate. The study is expected to report in the spring of 2018 for phase 1 and 2022 for phase 2.

Endo-bronchial coils:

Coils are nitinol wires with a predetermined shape (figure 27). They are inserted through a leading catheter. The 'birth-shape' is formed inside the bronchial tree. An average 10 coils are inserted in each lobe (figure 28) aiming at treating two lobes. The treatment is normally bilateral with 1-4 months separation time between the two procedures. Coils are permanent devices that are not reversible or removable once inserted. It is thought that coils act by 3 mechanisms:

1. Volume reduction by folding lung tissues.
2. Increasing elastic recoil of the emphysematous areas
3. Supporting small and medium size airways that are likely to collapse during expiration.

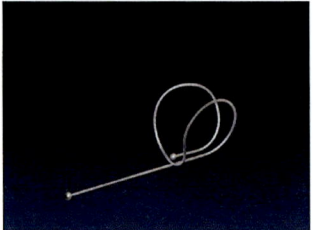 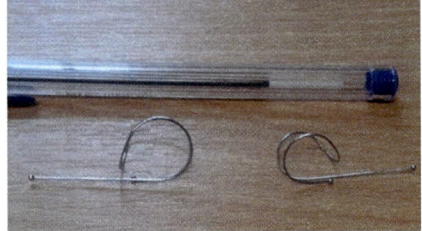

Figure 27: Endo-bronchial coil – Two coils compared to a size of a writing pen.

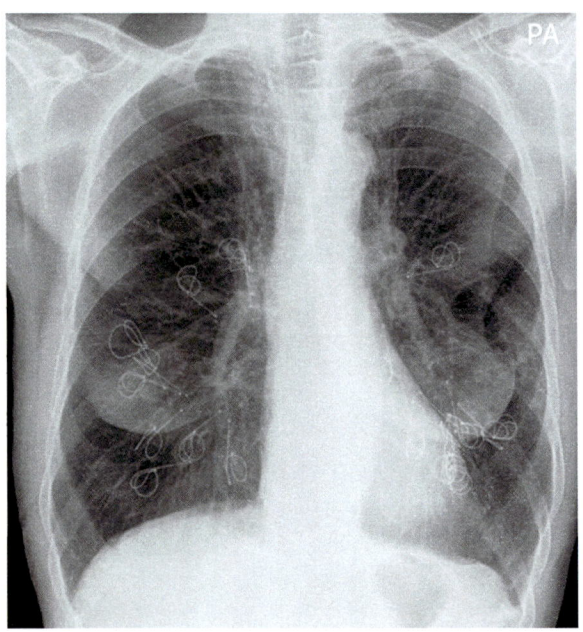

Figure 28: Bilateral coils inserted in the two lower lobes

Coils are inserted under image intensifier (figure 29) under heavy sedation or general anaesthesia. The efficacy of the coil is not affected by the absence of collateral ventilation or by the degree of heterogeneity of emphysema.

Several open feasibility studies found that coil insertion was safe. These were reported by Herth 2010, Selbos 2012, Klooster 2014 and Deslee 2014. In the first randomised prospective trial by Shah (2013) et al

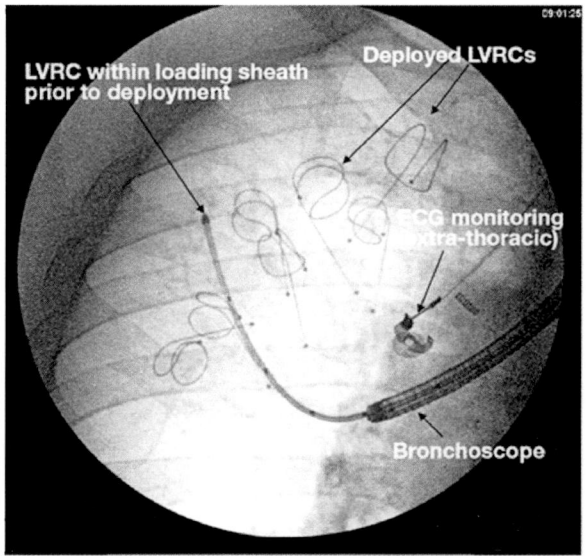

Figure 29: Lung volume reduction coils (LVRC) are inserted under the direction of image intensifier (direct vision fluoroscopy).

(the RESET trial) described benefit of endo-bronchial coils after three months in patients with homogeneous and heterogeneous emphysema. In the 47 patients recruited 23 received coil treatment. The main aim of the study was improvement of subjective markers using the SGRQ.

The study found a significant improvement at SGRQ in the coil group after ninety days. The study also reported improvement in other secondary outcome measures. The main adverse events occurred in the first months. This included two pneumothoraces and increase in the rate of exacerbations. Between 30-90 days, no adverse events were described.

The effect of coil in patients going into the RESET trial was re-examined twelve months after coil insertion (Zoumot 2015). Reduced efficacy was seen in all study end points. However, the improvement of benefit remains clinically significant for SGRQ, Residual Volume and for FEV1 and 6-MWD. The study found similar benefit in homogeneous and heterogeneous emphysema.

Similar findings were reported in a pan-European prospective, open label twelve months study (Deslee 2014).

Two large prospective clinical trials using endo bronchial coils were recently described. The first was performed in France - the REVOLENS study (2016) and the second was conducted in the US- the RENEW study.

The REVOLENS study recruited one hundred patients from ten French Hospitals. The aim of the study was to investigate efficacy (by looking at 6-MWD), side effects and economical value of endo-bronchial coils. The study found a significant improvement of 6-MWD, FEV1 and SGRQ in the coil group compared to those with usual care. This improvement was maintained for a year. There was a slight increase in adverse effect in the coil group with regards to pneumothoraces and COPD exacerbations. There were four deaths in the coil group and three in the usual care arm.

Several shortcomings were reported for the REVOLENS study. Significant improvement was due to decline in these parameters in the control group rather than improvement in the coil group. Patients were included without standardisation of the CT scan and finally patients on oxygen therapy (60% of patients) were not allowed oxygen during the 6-MW test.

The RENEW study (Scuirba 2016) is the largest clinical trial of coils to date. The trial recruited 315 patients with randomisation rate of 1:1. The main end-point of the study was the difference in 6 MWD at twelve months between coil insertion and standard care. Half way through the study, inclusion criteria were extended to include patients with less hyper-inflation (RV over 175% of expected values).

The study reported a modest improvement in primary end-point for all patients. Between the group difference was 14.6 m in 6-MWD in favour of the coil with 40 % achieving the 26 m – minimal clinically improvement difference. The improvement of SGRQ was more significant with a mean between-the-group difference of -8.9 points in favour of the coil group.

A subgroup analysis found greater benefit from coil treatment measured by several end points with hyper-inflation (Residual volume of 225% predicted). The discussion of the study however pointed out that a cut-off point of 200% of predicted was a better discriminator for likely responders.

For the first time the study distinguished between post coil pneumonia and post coil reaction to the tension induced by insertion of several coils. The studies demonstrated that those with post coil consolidation tended to respond more favourably and for a long period of time to coil insertion.

Further analysis found that when coils were inserted bilaterally into the lobes most affected with emphysema by QCT scans, the objective and subjective benefits significantly increased (Shah 2017 – American Thoracic Society Conference – Washington DC).

Sclerosing agents:

Sclerosing agents (hot steam and air seal polymers) have been tested in emphysema. The two methods create lung inflammations in the treatment site that would result in localised fibrosis followed by volume reduction.

Prospective studies investigating safety and efficacy have been done for both agents.

- *Hot water vapour- Steam:*

This procedure uses thermal energy from heated water vapour (figure 30) to induce inflammation followed by lung fibrosis which leads to volume reduction in the treated area (figure 31).

The obvious concern is that this procedure can result in uncontrolled inflammation manifested with pneumonia-like symptoms of fever, breathlessness, haemoptysis, chest pain and fatigue.

The first study to report benefit of the steam therapy was published by Snell et al in 2012. This was an open label study of forty-four patients run in two centres in Australia and Europe. Patients had severe predominantly upper lobe emphysema. At six months there was improvement in most lung function tests and in all components of SGRQ. In addition, there was an impressive volume loss averaged over 700 ml in the treated lobes.

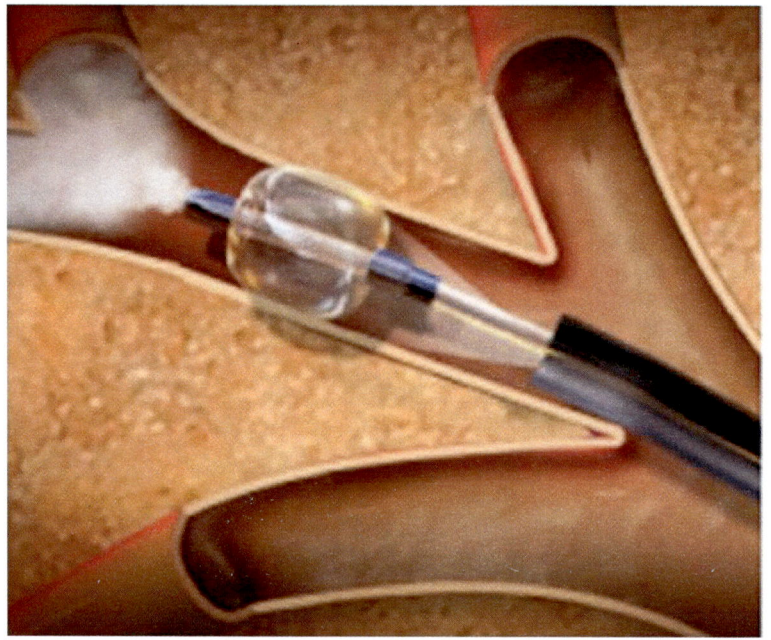

Figure 30: A schematic presentation of the water vapour deployment system

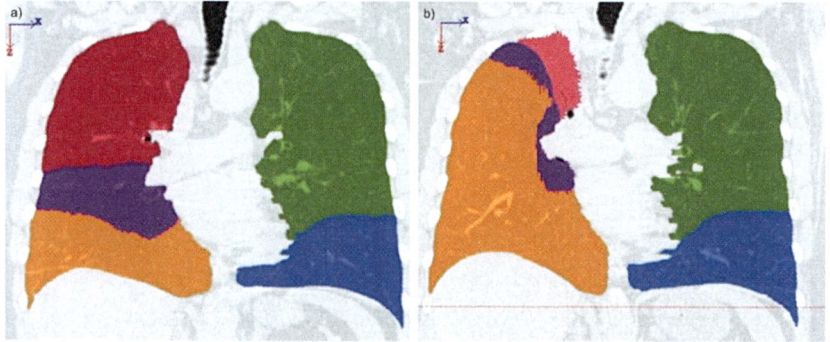

Figure 31: A coronal CT scan of lung lobes before (left) and 6-months after (right) of treatment of the right upper lobe with single episode of water vapour treatment. Note the loss of volume in the right upper lobe and the expansion in volume of the right lower lobe. From Snell et al (2012)

Significant side effects were noted, but all were predictable. These included pneumonic symptoms of cough, fever, chest pain and haemoptysis. Death occurred in only one patient, sixty-seven days from receiving water vapour treatment.

A further trial (STEP-UP) trial was reported in 2016 (Herth 2016). This was a 2:1 randomised trial in patients with highly heterogeneous emphysema and upper lobe predominant disease. Notably, in this trial, hot water vapour was instilled in the target lobe at two stages three months apart. At the second stage up to two segments were treated. Calculation of tissue-to-air ratio was made on HRCT scan to work out the amount of vapour needed to deliver. The main two end points were change in FEV1 and SGRQ.

A total of 134 patients were included. At six months the study achieved all its end points. FEV1 improved by 14.7%, residual volume decreased by 300 ml and SGRQ score decreased by 9.7 points. Clinically important difference was seen in 50% of all patients receiving steam compared to 13% in the control arm. Increased inflammatory symptoms were seen in the 18% vs 8% in the treatment groups with one death three months after treatment with water steam. One of the initial shortcomings of

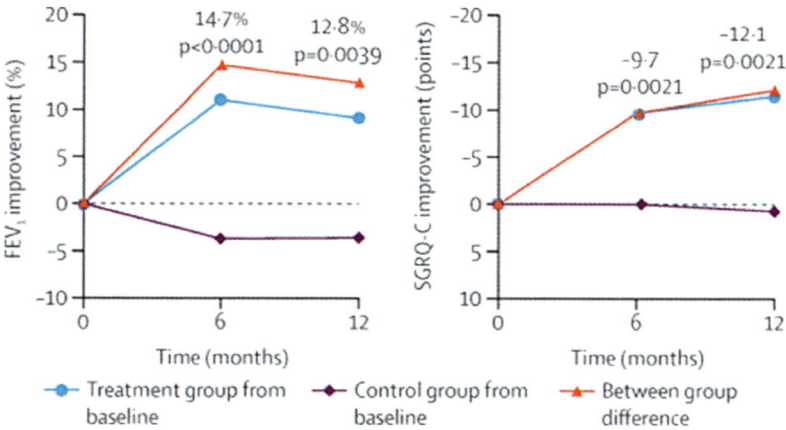

Figure 32: Improvement of FEV1 and SGRQ at 6 months and 12 months after sequential treatment with water vapour. Hearth 2016 (for the 6 months) – and Shah 2016 (for the 12 months results)

the STEP-UP trial was in its design. For a trial where the subjective SGRQ is one of its components, a group receiving sham procedure would strengthen the findings of the study.

A follow-up letter to the Lancet Respiratory Medicine, Shah et al (2016) reported that the benefit of the treatment extended to twelve months following the treatment (figure 32). More work needs to be done in patients with lower lobe disease. The number and intensity of treatment needs to be evaluated. The benefit-risk analysis needs to be further evaluated. However, given the fact that water is the only agent used, this treatment is very promising and may be used on a wider scale worldwide.

- *Aeri-Seal foam treatment:*

The Aeri-Seal system introduces a polymer material to the small airways and alveoli. The material is thought to function by preventing air entering the alveoli, closing inter-lobar collateral channels and create a film on the surface of the alveoli and the small airways. At a later stage an inflammatory process ensues that result in volume reduction (Figure 33).

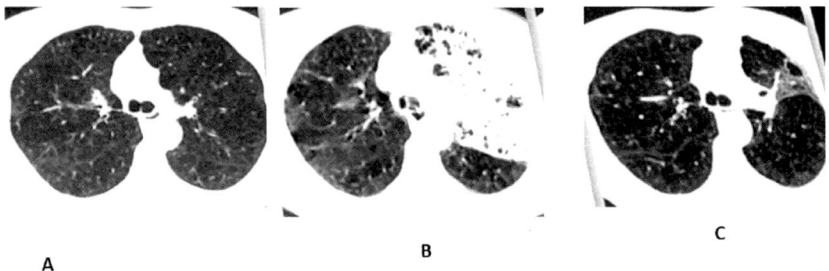

Figure 33: Three CT scans of a patient treated with Aeri-Seal *in the left upper lobe.*
A. Before the treatment
B. 3-weeks after treatment showing pneumonic changes
C. 3-months after treatment showing volume reduction in the treated lobe with fibrosis.

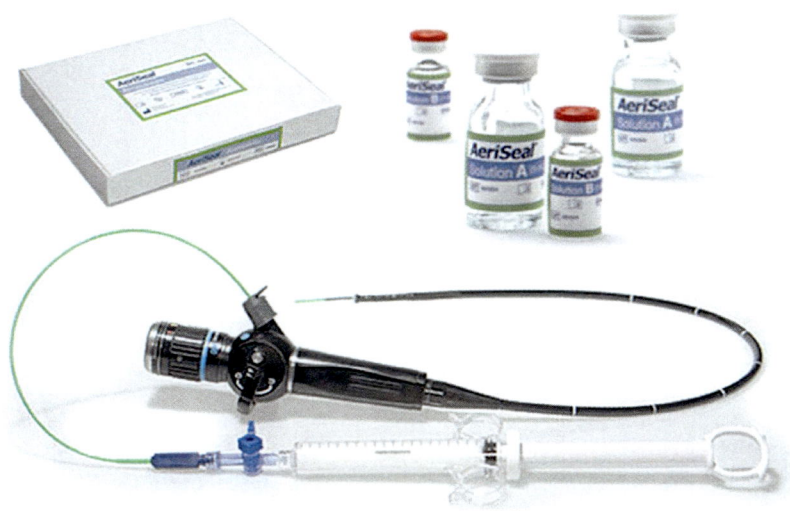

Figure 34: The set used to inject Aeri-Seal. *The two materials are known as solution a and b. The mixing syringe and the catheter are used in deployment of the mixed solution. The injection needs to be done within less than 60 seconds from completion of the mixing process.*

The material used is a combination of aminated polyvinyl alcohol, glutaraldehyde and air. The mixing process needs to happen quickly and so is the introduction of the foamy material through a catheter to the target area (figures 34). Unlike water vapour, where the inflammatory reaction occurs few days to weeks from the treatment, signs of respiratory symptoms in the Aeri-Seal occur within twenty-four hours.

The ASPIRE study was designed to investigate prospectively the Aeri-Seal in patients with upper lobe emphysema. The trial aimed at recruiting 300 patients. The study had to be terminated after involving only 95 patients due to lack of financial resources. The physicians involved in the study, took it upon themselves to analyse the data available at three and six months.

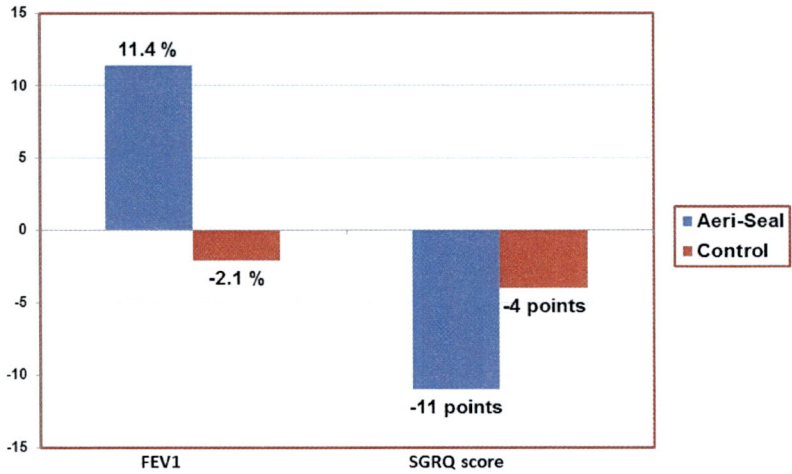

Figure 35: Change in FEV1 and SGRQ after at 3 months after Aeri-Seal insertion. The results persisted at the 6 months point. (Come CE 2016.)

Most of the analyses were limited due to the small number of patients. Data from the first three months are seen in figure 35. Data at six months was available on only twenty-one patients. Nevertheless, a clinically significant improvement in FEV1, 6-MWD and SGRQ was seen in 18%, 18% and 72% respectively.

Two deaths occurred in the treatment group and inflammatory adverse effects were seen in 44% of the candidates.

More recently the right of ownership has been bought by PulmonX (the owner of the Zephyr endo-bronchial valve) who are undertaking steps for multicentre, placebo control trials on a treatment approach that involve small doses of AeriSeal over several treatment periods in a similar way to the STEP-UP trial for water vapour.

Heterogeneous versus homogeneous emphysema

Unlike the previous thinking, it is rarely that we see totally homogeneous emphysema. Modern HRCT scans and particularly quantitative HRCT scans usually show heterogeneity. Heterogeneity of emphysema is defined as the difference in lung destruction between two adjacent lobes.

The cut-off point which defines homogeneous and heterogeneous emphysema is not clear. The LIBERATE trial defined heterogeneity of 15% difference between the target lobe and the adjacent lobe.

Clinical trials showing useful results for endo-bronchial valves and endo bronchial coils with less heterogeneity present. Valipour et al (2015) reported that in the IMPACT study an improvement in FEV1 and SGRQ in patients with 'homogeneous' emphysema (2015). Kemp et al (American Thoracic Society Meeting May 2017- not published as a manuscript yet) demonstrated further improvement in almost all subjective and objective parameters in the TRANSFORM Study where heterogeneity was less than 15%.

The Stelvio study (Klooster 2015) also compared the efficacy of endobronchial valves in homogeneous and heterogeneous emphysema using the 15% difference as a distinguisher. The study found that valves were useful in both, but more so in heterogeneous emphysema.

For coil insertion, the RENEW Study found no difference according to homogeneity of the disease. Therefore, the concept of heterogeneity of emphysema has lost its impact on patient's selection. For valve insertion it is the absence of collateral ventilation that is important. For coil insertion, it is the greater residual volume and the insertion of coils in the most destructed lobes that matter.

The optimal outcome of volume reduction therapies:

Various clinical trials of methods of lung volume reduction therapies used different main outcome. Valve trial all used FEV1 as the main outcome. Other objective outcome measures were used.

Study	Year	Device	Primary outcome
VENT	2010	Valve	FEV1
RESET	2013	Coil	QoL (St George's)
Stelvio (2015), IMPACT (2016) and LIBERATE (ongoing)	2018	Valve	FEV1
RENEW	2016	Coil	6' walk distance
Deslee (European Trial)	2014	Coil	QoL St George's
NETT	2003	Surgery	Exercise capacity- Survival
Believer HiFi	2013	Valve	FEV1
Coil European Registry Study	2018	Coil	QoL St George's
STEP-UP Trial	2016	Thermal vapour	FEV1 & St George's

Figure 36: A table showing outcome used in large clinical trials. Note that FEV1 was the main outcome in all valve studies but in none of the studies investigated using other methods of treatment.

These included reductions in residual volume and the 6-MWD. Subjective measures such as health related quality of life, mainly SGRQ was also used.

Surgical trials including the NETT trial used survival as the main outcome. Non-valve studies used 6-MWD for coils and SGRQ for steam as the principal outcome. Composite outcome including BODE score was used in one analysis as a surrogate marker for survival (Valipour 2014).

Outcome used in trials published thus far is outlined in figure 36.

It is the author's belief that, for future studies, one objective assessment and one subjective assessment should be used for all methods as the main outcome.

References

- Abboud RT and Vimalanathan S. Pathogenesis of COPD. Part I. The role of protease-antiprotease imbalance in emphysema [State of the Art Series]. Chronic obstructive pulmonary disease in high- and low-income countries. Int J Tuberc Lung Dis 2008; 12(4): 361–367.

- Brantigan OC, Mueller E, Kress MB. A surgical approach to pulmonary emphysema. Am Rev Respir Dis 1959; 80:194.

- Celli BR, Cote CG, Marin JM, Casanova C. The Body mass index, airflow limitation, dyspnoea and exercise capacity index in chronic obstructive pulmonary disease. N Eng J Med 2004; 350: 1005-1012.

- Cooper JD, Trulock EP, Triantafillou AN, et al. Bilateral pneumectomy (volume reduction) for chronic obstructive pulmonary disease. J Thorac Cardiovasc Surg 1995;109:106–16.

- Come CE, Kramer MR, Dransfield MT, et al. A randomised trial of lung sealant versus medical therapy for advanced emphysema. Eur Respir J 2015; 46: 651–62

- Criner GJ, Cordova FC, Furukawa S, et al. Prospective randomized trial comparing bilateral lung volume reduction surgery to pulmonary rehabilitation in severe chronic obstructive pulmonary disease. Am J Respir Crit Care Med 1999; 160:2018–27.

- Davey C, Zoumot Z, McNulty WH, Jordan S, Carr D et al. Bronchoscopic lung volume reduction with endo-bronchial valves for patients with heterogeneous emphysema and intact inter-lobar fissures (BeLieVeR-HIFi): a randomised controlled trial. Lancet 2015; 386: 1066-1073.

- Deslée G, Klooster K, Hetzel M et al. Lung volume reduction coil treatment for patients with severe emphysema: a European multicentre trial. Thorax.2014;69 (11):980-986.

- Deslée G, Mal H, Dutau H et al; REVOLENS Study Group. Lung volume reduction coil treatment vs usual care in patients with severe emphysema: the REVOLENS randomized clinical trial. JAMA. 2016;315(2):175-184.

- Diaz AA, Valim C, Yamashiro T, Estépar RS, Ross JC, Matsuoka S, Bartholmai B, Hatabu H, Silverman EK, Washko GR. Airway count and emphysema assessed by chest CT imaging predicts clinical outcome in smokers. Chest 2010; 138:880-887.

- Geddes D, Davies M, Koyama H, et al. Effect of lung-volume-reduction surgery in patients with severe emphysema. N Engl J Med 2000; 343:239–45.

- Global Strategy for the diagnosis, management and prevention of COPD, Global initiative for Chronic Obstructive Pulmonary Disease (GOLD 2016). http://www.goldcopd.org/- accessed October 2016.

- Goddard PR, Nicholson EM, Laszlo G, Watt I. Computed tomography in pulmonary emphysema. Clin Radiol 1982; 33:379-387.
- Gompelmann D, Eberhardt R, Ernst A, et al. The localized inflammatory response to bronchoscopic thermal vapor ablation. Respiration 2013; 86: 324–31. 32
- Gompelmann D, Herth FJF, Slebos DJ, Valipour A, Ernst A, Criner GJ, Eberhardt R. Pneumothorax following endo-bronchial valve therapy and impact on clinical outcomes in severe emphysema. Respiration 2014; 87: 485–491.
- Hartman JE, Klooster K, Gortzak K, Ten Hacken NH, Slebos DJ. Long-term follow-up after bronchoscopic lung volume reduction treatment with coils in patients with severe emphysema. Respirology 2015; 20: 319–26.
- Herth FJ, Gompelmann D, Stanzel F, et al. Treatment of advanced emphysema with emphysematous lung sealant (AeriSeal(R)). Respiration 2011; 82: 36–45. 34
- Herth FJ, Noppen M, Valipour A. Efficacy predictors of lung volume reduction with Zypher valves in a European Cohort. Eur Respir J 2012; 39: 1334-1342.
- Herth FJF, Eberhardt R, Gomplemann D, Ficker JH et al. Radiological and clinical outcomes of using ChartisTM to plan endobronchial valve treatment. Eur Respir J 2013; 41: 302-308.
- Herth FJ, Valipour A, Shah PL, et al. Segmental volume reduction using thermal vapour ablation in patients with severe emphysema: 6-month results of the multicentre, parallel-group, open-label, randomised controlled STEP-UP trial. Lancet Respir Med 2016; 4: 185–93. 33
- Herzog D, Thomsen C, Poellinger A, Doellinger F et al. Outcome of endobronchial valve treatment based on the precise criteria of an endobronchial catheter for detection of collateral ventilation under spontaneous breathing. Respiration 2016; 91 (1): 69-78.
- Hillerdal G, Löfdahl CG, Ström K, Skoogh BE, Jorfeldt L et al. Comparison of lung volume reduction surgery and physical training on health status and physiologic outcomes: a randomized controlled clinical trial. Chest. 2005 Nov;128(5):3489-99.
- Hopkinson NS, Kemp SV, Toma TP, et al. Atelectasis and survival after bronchoscopic lung volume reduction for COPD. Eur Respir J 2011; 37: 1346–51
- Klooster K, Ten Hacken NH, Franz I, Kerstjens HA, van Rikxoort EM, Slebos DJ. Lung volume reduction coil treatment in chronic obstructive pulmonary disease patients with homogeneous emphysema: a prospective feasibility trial. Respiration 2014;88 (2):116-125.
- Klooster K, Ten Hacken NHT, Hartman J.E, Kerstjens HAM, et al. Endo-bronchial Valves for Emphysema without Inter-lobar collateral ventilation. N Eng J Med 2015; 373: 3325-3335.

- Klooster K, Hartman JE, Ten Hacken NHT, Slebos DJ. One year follow-up after endo-bronchial valve treatment in patients with emphysema without interlobar collateral ventilation. The STELVIO trial. American Thoracic Society Meetings 2016 – San Francesco.

- Koenigkam Santos M, Puderback M, Gompelmann D, Eberhardt R et al. Inclomplete Fissures in severe emphysematous patients evaluated with MDCT: Incidence and interobserver aagreement among radiologists and pneumologists. Eur J of Radiol 2012; 81: 4161-4166.

- Kontogianni K, Gerovasili V, Gompelmann D,et al. Effectiveness of endobronchial coil treatment for lung volume reduction in patients with severe heterogeneous emphysema and bilateral incomplete fissures: a six-month follow-up. Respiration.2014;88(1):52-60.

- McNulty W, Jordan S, Hopkinson NC on behalf of The British Thoracic Society. Attitudes and access to lung volume reduction surgery for COPD: a survey by the British Thoracic Society. BMJ Open Resp Research 2014;1:e000023. doi:10.1136/bmjresp-2014-000023.

- National Emphysema Treatment Trial Research Group. A Randomized Trial Comparing Lung-Volume–Reduction Surgery with Medical Therapy for Severe Emphysema. N Engl J Med 2003; 348:2059-2073

- Oliveira HG, Rambo R, Oliveira S , Macedo Neto AVD. Semi-Automated CT Fissure Integrity Assessment As A Guide To Decision Making In Bronchoscopic Emphysema Treatment Using One-Way Zephyr® Valves. Am J Crit Care Respi Med 2015; 191: A 1146

- Schroeder, JD, McKenzie As, Zach JA, Wilson CG et al. Relationships Between Airflow Obstruction and Quantitative CT Measurements of Emphysema, Air Trapping, and Airways in Subjects With and Without Chronic Obstructive Pulmonary Disease. Am J Radiol 2013; 201: 460-470.

- Schumann M, Raffy P, Yin Y, et al. Computed tomography predictors of response to endobronchial valve lung reduction treatment, comparison with Chartis. Am J Resp and Crit Care Med 2015, 191: 767-774.

- Sciurba F, Ernst A, Herth F, Strange C et al. A randomized study of endobronchial valves for advanced emphysema. N Engl J Med 2010; 363: 1233-1244

- Sciurba FC, Criner G, Strange C, Shah PL, et al. Effect of Endobronchial Coils vs Usual Care on Exercise Tolerance in Patients with Severe Emphysema The RENEW Randomized Clinical Trial. JAMA 2016; 315:2178-2189.

- Shah P, Herth FJF. Current Status of bronchoscopic lung volume reduction with endobronchial valves. Thorax 2014; 69: 280-286.

- Shah PL, Zoumot Z, Singh S, et al. Endobronchial coils for the treatment of severe emphysema with hyperinflation (RESET): a randomised controlled trial. Lancet

Respir Med 2013;1: 233–40

- Shah PL, Gompelmann D, Valipour A, McNulty W, et al. Letter to the Editor: Thermal vapour ablation to reduce segmental volume in patients with severe emphysema: STEP-UP 12 months results. Lancet Respiratory Medicine July 2016.
- Slebos DJ, Klooster K, Ernst A, Herth FJ, Kerstjens HA. Bronchoscopic lung volume reduction coil treatment of patients with severe heterogeneous emphysema. Chest.2012; 142(3): 574-582.
- Snell GI; Holsworth L; Borrill ZL; Thomson KR; at al. The Potential for Bronchoscopic Lung Volume Reduction Using Bronchial Prostheses: A Pilot Study. Chest 2003; 124 (3): 1073-1080.
- Snell GI, Herth FJF, Hopkins P, Baker KM et al. Bronchoscopic thermal vapour ablation therapy in the management of heterogeneous emphysema. Eur Respi J 2012; 39: 1326- 1333.
- Valipour A, Slebos DJ, de Oliveira HG, Eberhardt R, Freitag L, Criner GJ, Herth FJF. Expert Statement: Pneumothorax Associated with Endoscopic Valve Therapy for Emphysema – Potential Mechanisms, Treatment Algorithm, and Case Examples. Respiration 2014; 87:513–521.
- Valipour A, Herth FJF, Burghuber OC, Criner G et al. Target lobe volume reduction and COPD outcomes after endobronchial valve therapy. Eur Resp J 2014; 43: 387-396.
- Valipour A, Slebos D, Herth F et al. Endobronchial Valve Therapy in Patients with Homogeneous Emphysema. Results from the IMPACT Study. Am J Respir and Crit Care Med 2016; 194 (vol 1).
- Venuta F, Anile M, Diso D, Carilla C et al. Long-term follow-up after bronchoscopiclung volume reduction in patients with emphysema. Eur Respir J. 2012; 39: 1084-1089.
- Weder W, Tutic M, Lardinois D, Jungraithmayr W, Hillinger S, Russi EW, Bloch KE.Persistent benefit from lung volume reduction surgery in patients with homogeneous emphysema. Ann Thorac Surg. 2009 Jan;87(1):229-36.
- Zoumot Z, Kemp SV, Singh S, et al. Endobronchial coils for severe emphysema are effective up to 12 months following treatment: medium term and cross-over results from a randomised controlled trial. PLoS One 2015; 10: e0122656. 31

The Madhouses of St George

PETER CARPENTER

Presented at the Bristol Medico-Historical Society meeting on October19th 2016

England first developed widespread specialised care for the mentally ill in the 18th century with the growth of the madhouse business which blossomed in the early 19th Century before collapsing with the growth of the public lunatic asylum. These "madhouses" (as they were called at the time) were generally run by doctors but some were run by clerics and some by the doctors' widows. They were usually set up in large houses, in secluded places, and first regulated in 1774 when they had to be licenced and statistics start to be possible. Like any business they always had a unique selling point; usually about the individual skills of the proprietor, some advertising through books to broadcast their skills, as Mason Cox of Fishponds House did. When there were scandals the businesses suffered. When they did well they would move to larger premises or take over other asylums. There was a business and living to be made out of the madhouse trade!

In Bristol eight private madhouses were licenced – most created after 1800. Three of these survived to the 1950s, principally the larger purpose built places.

I'm going to talk about two less known in the St George area. Nowadays it is not a secluded rural situation but in the 1840s it was, as this map of 1880 shows (figure 1).

Whitehall House

Whitehall House is now demolished but gave its name to the area of Whitehall just north of St George. Whitehall House was probably over 100 years old by the time it became an asylum, and was the home of

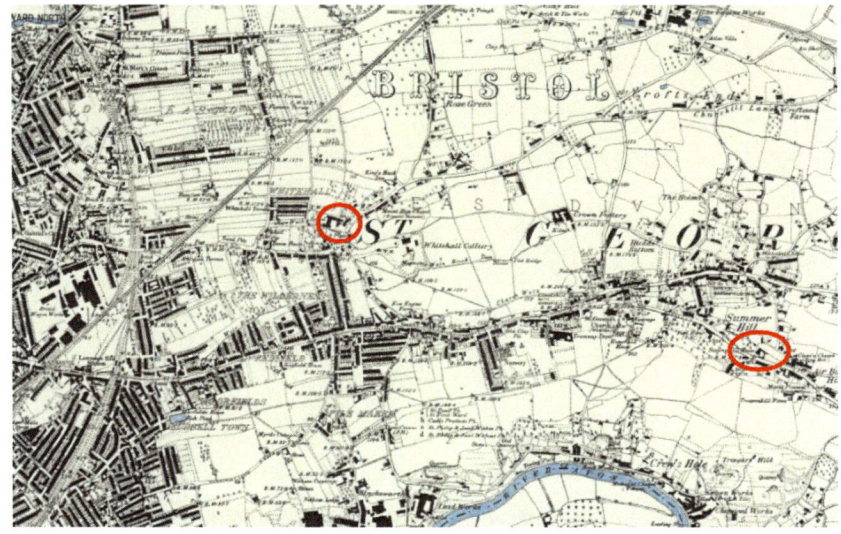

Figure 1. St George 1880 with sites of the two asylums marked

Henry Davis, banker, whose son Richard Hart Davis was member of parliament for Bristol from 1812 to 1831. After Henry died in 1804 and his widow in 1814, two of his daughters lived there until in 1829 they moved into a new house built next door – Woodbine Cottage. Whitehall House then put up for sale but stood empty looking for a use until it was rented by John Braithwaite Taylor in 1832 to be turned into an lunatic asylum for women.

John Braithwaite Taylor was the son of Major-General Aldwell Taylor of the East India Company, Madras. He was born in 1801 in the East, educated at St Pauls School and graduated as a physician from Edinburgh in 1824. He first worked in the Tewkebury Dispensary but then moved to Bristol where he offered lessons for medical students.

He rented Whitehall House in 1832 and in January applied to the Justices of the Peace for a licence to operate as a private asylum for up to twelve women with no pauper patients.

John first advertises the home in May 1832 as a private asylum and states he trusts in God's assistance in his work. At the same time he sent his prospectus around to local doctors and also the admission

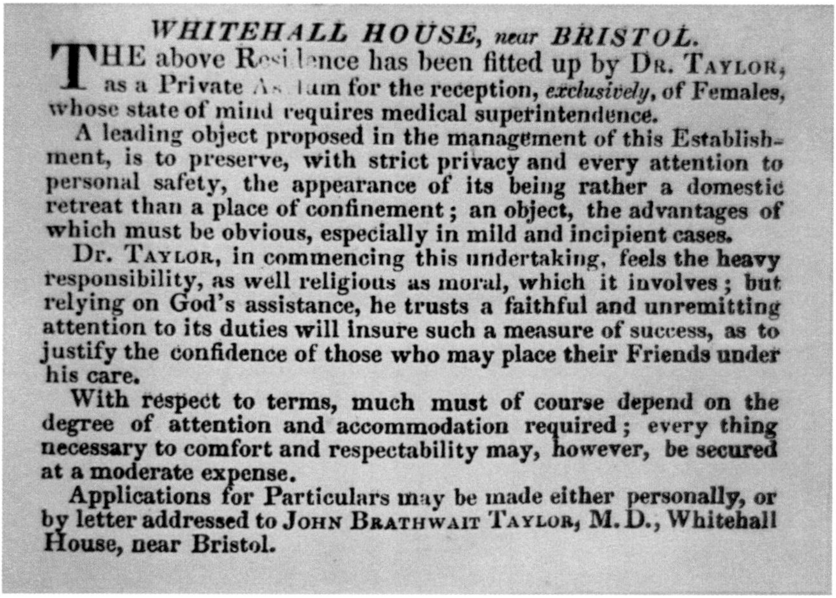

> **WHITEHALL HOUSE, near BRISTOL.**
>
> THE above Residence has been fitted up by Dr. Taylor, as a Private Asylum for the reception, *exclusively*, of Females, whose state of mind requires medical superintendence.
>
> A leading object proposed in the management of this Establishment, is to preserve, with strict privacy and every attention to personal safety, the appearance of its being rather a domestic retreat than a place of confinement; an object, the advantages of which must be obvious, especially in mild and incipient cases.
>
> Dr. Taylor, in commencing this undertaking, feels the heavy responsibility, as well religious as moral, which it involves; but relying on God's assistance, he trusts a faithful and unremitting attention to its duties will insure such a measure of success, as to justify the confidence of those who may place their Friends under his care.
>
> With respect to terms, much must of course depend on the degree of attention and accommodation required; every thing necessary to comfort and respectability may, however, be secured at a moderate expense.
>
> Applications for Particulars may be made either personally, or by letter addressed to John Brathwait Taylor, M.D., Whitehall House, near Bristol.

Figure 2 Advert for the opening of Whitehall [Bristol Mirror 26 May 1832]

certificates that needed to be completed for patients to be admitted legally.

Interestingly though soon after the start he also extends his potential by offering himself as a candidate for the vacant medical position at St Peter's Hospital, saying that his conduct of Whitehall House makes him a suitable candidate.

When you look at the patient numbers you realise that these were chronic patients with a slow turn over - there are only three patients admitted in the first year and seven in the next of whom one dies and four are removed.

John Taylor died in 1833. He had married Martha Ann Parsons, the daughter of a English army captain. She took over the business until she died in 1848, initially with a Mr Shorland visiting as surgeon, but later with her brother John Dungate Featherstonhaugh Parsons. John Parsons was born in Ireland in 1814 when his family were stationed out there.

The plans put in for the original licensing show a fairly unremarkable four-storey house. It is unclear how it would be used as an asylum but this becomes slightly clearer in a revised plan one year later which shows the third attic floor converted into five bedroom cells and the second floor with bedrooms and sitting rooms.

By 1841 Martha is living there with her four children, eight patients, four female servants and her brother John Parsons. Interestingly the house is put up for sale again by the Davis family in 1844 and may have been bought by the Taylors. By 1847 they got to ten patients but then Martha died from a *'Visitation of God'* in 1848. The business was continued by her brother John Parsons who had married John Taylor's sister Jane.

John Parsons clearly decided that he wanted to expand and applied for extensions to the buildings with twelve more bedrooms which he then built.

The census return of 1851 shows him with his wife and two of Martha's younger orphan children, with nine female inmates all of whom are gentlewomen though one is also stated to the daughter of a baronet and another of a naval officer. Interestingly only two female lunatic attendants live in with a cook and general servant, suggesting that the work was not onerous or dangerous.

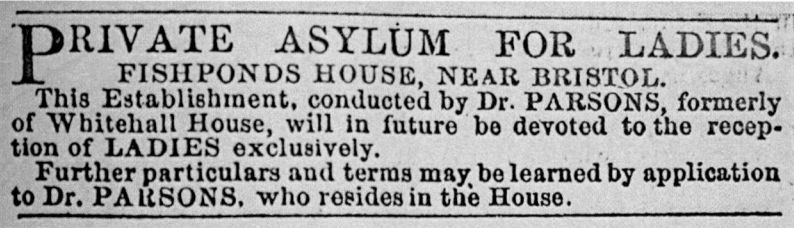

Figure 3
1855 Advertisement for Fishponds House

Fishponds Asylum

During 1849 to 1851 the nearby large Fishponds Asylum was going from one disaster to another with public scandals about care followed by changes of management and the injection of money to improve its fabric followed by the unexpected death of the new manager. John

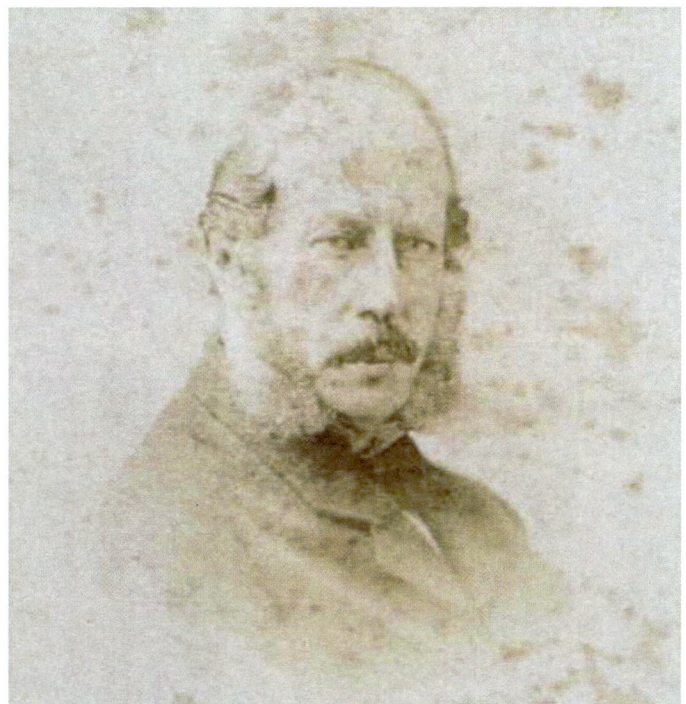

Figure 4. John Dungate Featherstonhaugh Parsons in his later years

Parsons appears to have seized his opportunity and even though he had only just enlarged Whitehall, took over the larger and well adapted Fishponds House. Whitehall House was put up for sale with its new three story extension but failed to sell and became derelict until it was demolished and the site used for Whitehall School. The lane by it was called Madhouse Lane until it was renamed Bourneville Road in the 20th Century.

When Parsons moved with his patients he moved from looking after ten women to nine men and twenty-two women. He seems to have decided to go back to women only and advertised this in 1855.

Rather usefully in 1854 he described his views on treatment to the Commmissioners:

'Mechanical restraint is never employed, except when it may become necessary in the course of surgical treatment, to prevent, for instance, the forcible removal of dressings from a wound. One instance of this has

occurred during the last two years. Seclusion is scarcely more frequently resorted to, only one patient having been subjected to it within the year.

In the medical treatment of acute mania, as well as of the paroxysms of excitement and violence which occur in chronic cases, I rely chiefly on the use of narcotics and sedatives (opium, morphia and hyoscyamus), with purgatives, and the warm bath and cold shower-bath.

Bleeding, either general or topical, ought not, I think to be reckoned among the remedies for any form of insanity. Indeed the coexistence of insanity with any other disease which may call for bleeding makes me more than usually cautious in the use of it.

Nauseates, as a means of subduing excitement, I am not in the habit of prescribing. I have had several patients under my care to whom they have previously been given, whose mental and bodily condition has certainly improved since they have ceased to take them.'

John Parsons seems to have planned to continue in the Lunacy Business. In 1856 he negotiated a fourteen year lease of Fishponds House from the owners, the Bompas family.

But he then had problems with the Commissioners in Lunacy who told him to tell relatives to remove two of his patients to other establishments as they felt they would do better if moved. John Parsons did this but the people were not removed and there is then conflict over the next years where the Commissioners put mounting pressure on him to have the patients moved including using the local magistrates. The magistrates are sympathetic to John and comments that John Parsons acted under trying circumstances and had been suffering from severe gout to explain his brusque manner but they bemoan the fact that the commissioners were basically branding his asylum as inferior to some others. Interestingly the two patients did move but appear to have died soon after. The next year, in 1859, Fishponds House is put up for sale. John Parsons moved to Dowry Square and went into work in general practice including at the Clifton Dispensary.

Summerhill House

The other place I talked about is that operated by Thomas Dowling Eyre in Summerhill House. He was the fourth child of six children of the Rev William Eyre of Wells who married Charlotte Dowling of

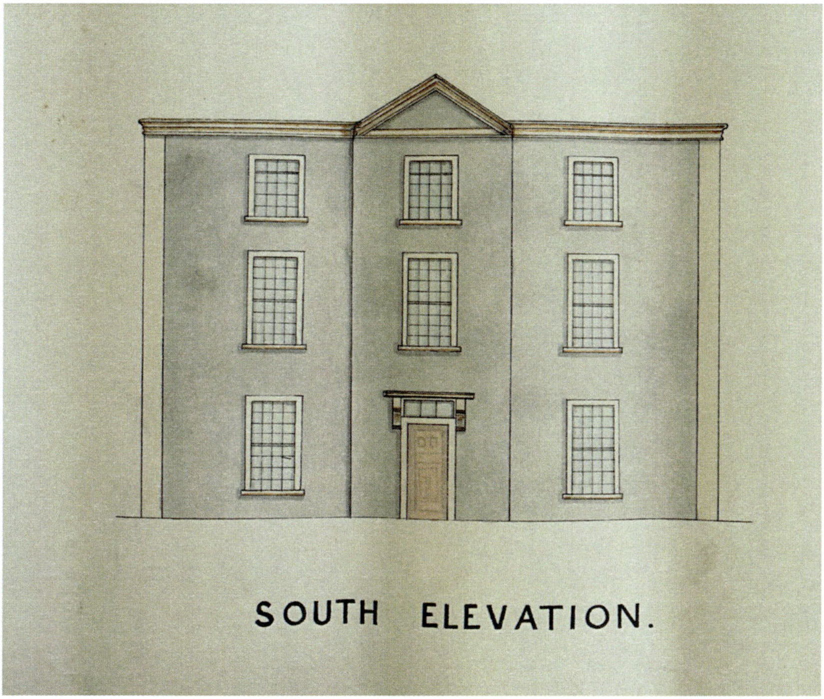

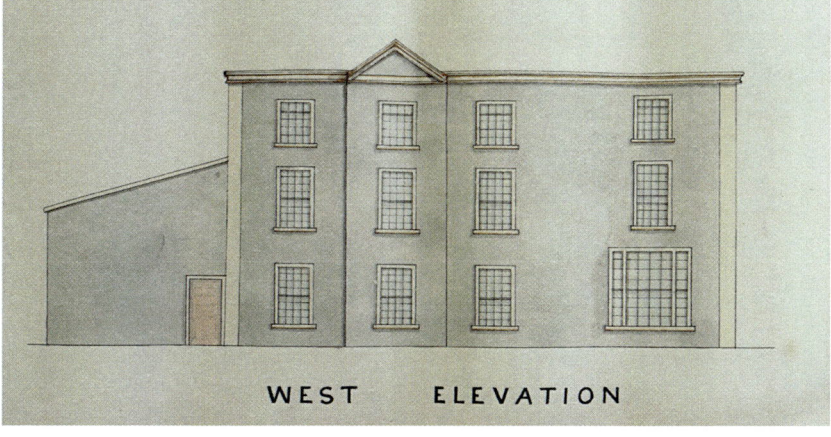

Figures 5a and 5b
Images of Summerhill House from the licence Application.

Chew Magna in 1790. He was born in 1795 and married his cousin Mary Dowling who was the daughter of Joseph Dowling surgeon in Chew Magna. He himself is stated in a family tree to have been a Captain in the Royal Marines and I cannot find evidence that he was a surgeon – he is always referred to as 'gentleman'.

In 1841 he is living with his wife with his widowed mother Charlotte in her house, Summerhill House. With them appear to be two or three other families they are probably renting rooms to.

In 1843 he applies for a £15 annual licence for Summerhill House to become a lunatic asylum for up to three men. However he never seems to have more than two men in it and in 1849 surrenders the licence to have only one patient which meant that he no longer needed to pay out £15 for the licence. To be an asylum he needed a visiting surgeon and this may have been his brother in law, Thomas Dowling of Chew Magna.

In 1851 he is there with his wife and two servants and one patient, John Stokes aged seventy-six from London along with his attendant James who is aged twenty, from Wiltshire.

In September 1858 Mr Eyre tries to sell Summerhill House. He died two years later of stomach cancer and his will notes effects of under £1000. His widow moved back Chew Magna to live with her brother Thomas Dowling the GP there and she died fifteen years later.

Summerhill House itself was a fairly non-descript house set by the road at Summer Hill just before one reaches Air Balloon Hill. There seems nothing remarkable about it except I note it had eleven bedrooms. It was demolished in the 1960s and is now covered by modern Housing.

Acknowlegements

I am grateful to Dr Peter Parsons, descendant of the Whitehall House Proprietors, for his material on the people and asylum and image of JDF Parsons. The plans of the houses are at the Gloucestershire Archives, for whom I am grateful for the images of Summerhill House. Fishponds asylum is well described by Dr H Temple Phillips in his thesis *"The History of the old private lunatic asylum at Fishponds, Bristol"*.

The Lives of Two Pioneering Medical-Chemists in Bristol
Thomas Beddoes (1760-1808)
and William Herapath (1796-1868)

Brian Vincent

School of Chemistry, University of Bristol, Bristol, BS8 1TS.

Presented at the meeting on Dec 12th 2016

ABSTRACT

From the second half of the 18th century onwards the new science of chemistry took root and applications were heralded in many medical-related fields, e.g. cures for diseases such as TB, the prevention of epidemics like cholera, the application of anaesthetics and the detection of poisons in forensics. Two pioneering chemists who worked in the city were Thomas Beddoes, who founded the Pneumatic Institution in Hotwells in 1793, and William Herapath who was the first professor of chemistry and toxicology at the Bristol Medical School, located near the Infirmary, which opened in 1828. As well as their major contributions to medical-chemistry, both men played important roles in the political life of the city.

INTRODUCTION

The second half of the 18th century saw chemistry emerge as a fledgling science. Up till then there was little understanding of the true nature of matter. The classical Greek idea that matter consisted of four basic elements (earth, fire, water and air) still held sway, as did the practice of alchemy: the search for the *"elixir of life"* and for the *"philosophers' stone"* which would turn base metals into gold. Also, the *"phlogiston"* theory of fire was still to the forefront. This idea proposed that when any material, such as wood, burnt an integral component, phlogiston, was released.

The new thinking originated with the discovery that *"air"* was not a single substance, as previously supposed, but rather was made of a mixture of different substances. Leading the way were a group of British scientists, starting with Joseph Black in Glasgow, who isolated carbon dioxide from air in the early 1750s; one of his pupils, Daniel Rutherford, discovered nitrogen in 1772. The Yorkshireman, Joseph Priestley is generally credited with discovering oxygen in 1774. He went on to discover several other gases including carbon monoxide, sulphur dioxide, and nitrous and nitric oxides. Meanwhile Henry Cavendish, in London, had discovered hydrogen in 1766. Moreover, Antoine Lavoisier, in Paris in the late 1770s, showed that combustion involves the material concerned combining with oxygen, thus demolishing the phlogiston theory.

In the medical field, physicians and apothecaries, at that time, still prescribed for the most part long-established, natural drugs based largely on plant extracts. This article tells the story of two pioneering chemists in Bristol who developed their research and medical practice around the new, emerging science of chemistry: Thomas Beddoes and William Herapath. Since Herapath was only twelve when Beddoes died, it is unlikely that the two actually conversed. Nevertheless, they had much in common, not least that, as well as being scientists, they were both political dissenters and activists.

THOMAS BEDDOES (1760 - 1808)

Thomas Beddoes, the son of a wealthy tanner, was born in Shrifnal in Shropshire and was educated at Bridgnorth grammar school. In 1776 he went to Pembroke College, Oxford to study medicine. He also developed strong interests in botany, geology and languages. During the vacations Beddoes attended meetings

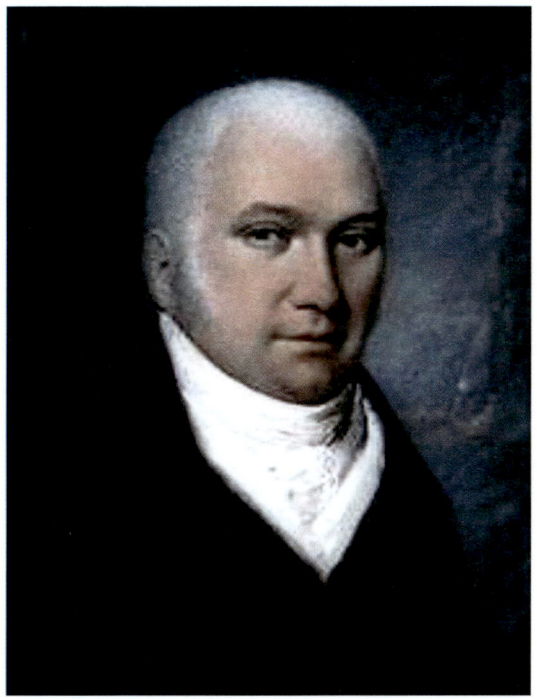

of the *"Lunar Society"*, which met in and around Birmingham. Here he would have met radical political and religious thinkers, such as Erasmus Darwin, Joseph Priestley, Josiah Wedgewood, James Watt & Matthew Boulton, William Reynolds, Richard Lovell Edgeworth and Joseph Wright.

After gaining his BA at Oxford in 1781, Beddoes moved to London to study anatomy with the famed teacher, Dr Sheldon. He moved back to Oxford in 1783 and took his MA degree. However, he decided to spend part of his time in Edinburgh in order to attend lectures in chemistry by Joseph Black (who by then had moved from Glasgow), since Beddoes, like Black, saw chemistry as the key to future developments in medicine. He gained his MD degree from Oxford in 1786. In the summer of 1787 he visited Antoine Lavoisier in Paris. Afterwards Beddoes took up an appointment as a reader in chemistry back at Oxford.

However, he was never really happy in this post. The facilities for his research were poor (a make-do lab in the bottom of the Ashmolean Museum) and the authorities (and increasingly his students also) took a dim view of his radical religious and political views – in particular his support for the revolution in France. Beddoes resigned his post in 1792.

Beddoes decided to move to Bristol, where his political and religious views would be more sympathetically received. He was particularly concerned with the plight of the poor, since tuberculosis and other contagious diseases were endemic in the new industrialised towns. Beddoes was keen to apply the new gases to try to treat such diseases.

In Hotwells the medical *"spa"* was long-established. So, in the spring of 1793, Beddoes opened a clinic (*the "Pneumatic Institution"*) at 11, Hope Square, Hotwells. Two of the patients who underwent the new gas treatment were Tom Wedgewood and Gregory Watt, the sons of two of his old Lunar Society friends: Josiah Wedgewood and James Watt. James Watt supplied Beddoes with some specially designed equipment for making and delivering the various gases.

Beddoes set up home in Clifton, at 3 Rodney Place. In 1794, he married the third daughter of Richard Lovell Edgeworth (a friend from Lunar Society days), Anna, who was thirteen years his junior. They had four children; their elder son, Thomas Lovell Beddoes (1803-1849) became one of the well-known, early 19th century romantic poets, although he moved to Germany in 1825. It was through Anna's elder sister, Maria, herself an author, that Beddoes became friends with three young poets then residing in Bristol: Robert Lovell, Robert Southey and Samuel Taylor Coleridge. Beddoes and Coleridge campaigned together in Bristol against slavery, in support (initially, at least) of the French Revolution and, in particular, against the so-called *"gagging bills"* which Prime Minister Pitt had introduced to suppress dissident political views.

For several years Beddoes had been trying to raise money to establish a bigger and better institution in Bristol, where he could further his research as well as treat patients. Eventually sufficient money was raised to open the new *"Pneumatic Institution"* at 6-7 Dowry Square in July 1799. At the suggestion of one of his former tutees at Oxford (and subsequent lifelong friend), Davies Giddy, then MP for Bodmin, Beddoes appointed a 19-year-old, precocious young man from Penzance, Humphry Davy, as the first superintendent of the new Institution. At Beddoes' suggestion, Davy started working on the gas nitrous oxide to see if it had any medical uses. Davy found it acted as a stimulant and mood enhancer, with strong psychedelic and hallucinogenic effects. Although Davy and Beddoes recognised it numbed pain they never sort to actually use it as an anaesthetic (that was to come later with Herapath). Instead it soon became used more as a "recreational" drug, which Davy shared with his new friends in Bristol; it was subsequently to become known as *"laughing gas"*.

By now the efficacy of Beddoes treatments was beginning to be questioned. Moreover, he had upset the local population somewhat. Firstly, he had set up a byre in Dowry Square to house cows, whose breath (rich in carbon dioxide) he thought might be used to treat tuberculosis patients. Secondly, there was the episode of the *"plague of frogs"*, when a consignment of these creatures he had ordered for some experiments escaped during unloading in the City docks.

In 1800, a new chemical passion caught Davy's imagination in Dowry Square: the use of Voltaic cells to produce gases by the process we now call electrolysis, in particular oxygen and hydrogen from water.

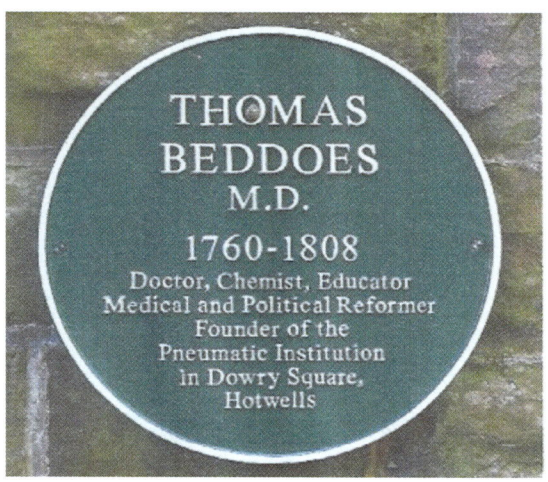

However, in 1801 Davy was *"poached"* by the recently established Royal Institution in London.

Thereafter Beddoes himself became increasingly more interested in promoting preventative medicine and health awareness amongst the poor in Bristol. He renamed his Dowry Square institute *"the Bristol Medical Institution"* and he opened a second practice in the midst of the city docks, on Broad Quay. He was very keen to see surgeons, apothecaries and physicians better trained. To this end, in 1797 he and two surgeons from the Bristol Infirmary (Francis Bowles & Richard Smith) started a course of popular lectures on anatomy, initially at the Red Lodge (on Park Row) and then at premises at 10, College Green. Bowles died of TB in 1800 and Beddoes' workload at the Medical Institution was increasing and so the course was abandoned.

The Bristol Medical Institution closed in 1807, after Beddoes himself became ill. He died on Dec 24 1808, aged 48. The autopsy showed that he had a collapsed left lung. He is buried in the Strangers Burial Ground off Lower Clifton Hill, where the plaque shown above may be found.

WILLIAM HERAPATH (1796-1868)

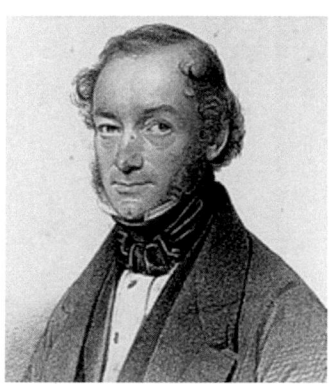

William Herapath was born Bristol in 1796 and was brought up for most of his childhood in the "Packhorse" public house in Lawrence Hill, which his father, originally from North Devon, ran, together with the associated brewery. When his father died in 1816 William inherited this thriving business, but he did not want to follow his father's profession. He was more interested in chemistry and began to develop an analytical chemistry practice working with local industries in and around Bristol. His first published paper in 1823 was concerned with the analysis of cadmium in zinc dust, work carried out in association with a local zinc smelting company.

Herapath married Sophia Bird in 1819 and they set up home initially at 56, Old Market Street and then at 2 Old Park, near St Michael's Hill. Like Beddoes, he was passionately interested in local and national politics. He was elected Vice President of the Bristol Political Union. He was very concerned about problems of public hygiene and campaigned strongly for public baths and washhouses. He also spoke out against the Bristol Corporation whom he thought were ineffective and corrupt.

When, in 1831, the House of Lords rejected the first reform bill, protests were held around the country. In Bristol these culminated in the infamous *"Bristol Riots"* which took place over the last weekend in October 1831. The mob attacked (and in many cases set fire to) various buildings in Bristol. Despite his antipathy towards the Corporation, Herapath, agreed to act as a *"special constable"* (along with Isambard Kingdom Brunel) at this time. He tried in vain to prevent the crowd from breaking down the gates of the new Bristol Gaol on Cumberland Road. The reform bill was finally passed in 1832 and Herapath served as a Liberal member on the newly reformed Bristol Corporation from 1835 to 1863. He also became a senior magistrate in Bristol.

All this political activity did not affect Herapath's medical and scientific work. In 1833 he was appointed as a lecturer (and subsequently professor) in chemistry and toxicology at the newly founded Bristol Medical School (located behind Park Row). He was a founding member of the Chemical Society (forerunner of the Royal Society of Chemistry) in London in 1841. He corresponded with many famous scientists, including Michael Faraday in London who requested a sample of cadmium from him.

Although anaesthetics had been used previously in London, in January 1847 Herapath was the first person in Bristol to administer a gas (ether) as a general anaesthetic during an operation; he assisted the surgeon during a leg amputation on a young man at the Bristol General Hospital. Herapath was very familiar with the work of Beddoes and Davy, and, a few days after this operation, he used nitrous oxide as a general anesthetic during a tooth extraction, again for the first time in Bristol.

Part of Herapath's role within the Bristol Medical School was as a chemical analyst. In this context he analysed the composition of the Hotwells spring water. He is, however, chiefly remembered for his work as a forensic chemical analyst. He was the first person to devise a definitive test for arsenic in a corpse. He gave evidence in many famous court cases involving poisoning. One of these was the trial at the Spring Assizes in Bristol in 1835 of Mary Ann Burdock, who was accused of murdering, by arsenic poisoning, Mrs Clara Ann Smith, a 60-year-old, relatively wealthy widow, who had been a lodger at the boarding house run by Mary Burdock in St Phillips. Mrs Smith's death in October 1833 was certified as being from *"natural causes"*. However, when in due course a nephew returned from overseas questions were asked: where was his inheritance and why had Mary Burdock apparently become so much richer? The upshot was that the coroner ordered an exhumation and autopsy of the body. Although the body had been in the grave for more than one year, Herapath was able to detect sufficient arsenic in the stomach to suggest poisoning. Mary Burdoch was arrested and on the evidence of Herapath and of a maid, who had observed Mary Burdoch administer a *"red powder"* to Mrs Smith, a remaining sample of which Herapath also showed contained arsenic, Mary Burdoch was convicted and subsequently hanged outside the new Bristol Gaol on Cumberland Road. A crowd, estimated to be 50,000 persons, gathered outside to witness the first public execution of a female at the gaol.

Herapath also appeared on occasions for the defence in murder trials. One such famous occasion was at the trial in 1855 at the Old Bailey in London of a doctor, William Palmer, in one of the most notorious cases of the 19th century. Palmer was arrested for the murder, allegedly by poisoning with strychnine, of his racing associate, John Cook. The police were also convinced he had murdered several other victims, including family members, for the life insurance money to feed his gambling habits on horses. In this case Herapath was up against some heavyweights. The lead barrister for the prosecution was the renowned and fearsome attorney general, Sir Alexander Cockburn, and the forensic witness called by the prosecution was Alfred Swain

Taylor, Professor of Medical Jurisprudence at Guys Hospital, who has been called *"The Father of Modern Toxicology"*. Herapath could find no evidence of strychnine in the body of John Cook. Ironically, Taylor could find none either! But the highly respected, London-based toxicologist stated that he was *"still convinced"* that Cook had been poisoned! Palmer was found guilty on purely circumstantial evidence and the biased summing up by the judge, Lord Chief Justice Campbell, who had also prevented Herapath from demonstrating his chemical test to the court. In 1859, on the basis of this and other cases, Herapath wrote a letter to The Times stating: *"I consider that professional witnesses, who give their opinions, where the life or freedom of a man is at stake, are as much on trial as the prisoner"*.

A major outbreak of cholera occurred in Bristol 1832, and then again in 1849. Herapath held the conventional view that cholera emanated from the putrid *"poison"*, associated with decaying animal flesh, which is inhaled into the lungs. He even suggested a chemical cure: fumigation with a mixture of black manganese oxide and common table salt, onto which vitriol (sulphuric acid) was poured. However, the real heroes in the fight against cholera in Bristol were a group of other doctors in the City (including William Budd, a doctor at the Infirmary, but also a director of the Waterworks company), who came to realize that cholera was not carried in the air, but in contaminated drinking water.

Herapath served as President of the *Bristol Philosophical and Literary Society*, at that time located on Park St. in what is now the Freemasons Hall. He was very interested in public education. In 1836 he delivered a series of four lectures on various scientific topics at the *Mechanics Institute* located in Broadmead: air and fire; water; cooking and brewing; and laughing gas. He repeated the laughing gas lecture at the *Bristol Philosophical and Literary Society* where hundreds were turned away! William Herapath retired from his post at the Medical School in 1867. He was a diabetic and died at home in February 1868 aged 71. His grave is in Arnos Vale Cemetery.

The Herapath family in Bristol established a minor scientific dynasty. William's cousin John Herapath (born 1790 in Bristol, but he later moved to London) was an applied mathematician and theoretical physicist. William's eldest son, William Bird Herapath FRS (born 1820), was both a surgeon and a scientist (he received his FRS for his discovery of the first light-polarising crystal, subsequently named *"herapathite"*). In addition, William's youngest son, Thornton John Herapath (born 1830) carried out some significant research as a chemical analyst, but sadly died when he was only twenty-eight. John Herapath's second son, Spencer (born 1821), became a civil engineer. The son, grandson and great-grandson of William Bird Herapath all became doctors in and around Bristol. So five, successive generations of the same family worked in the city as medical practitioners or scientists.

A plaque to Herapath

A plaque was erected in February 2017 by the Bristol Civic Society on the outside wall of the *"Packhorse"* pub in Lawrence Hill, where William Herapath lived prior to his marriage.

The only other commemoration to the Herapath family in Bristol is in nearby Barton Hill, where a road, "Herapath Street", was named in their honour.

BRISTOL CIVIC SOCIETY
Professor
William Herapath
1796 – 1868
Pioneering analytical and forensic
chemist and prominent
Bristol politician
Lived here
1800 – 1819

HERAPATH ST. BS5

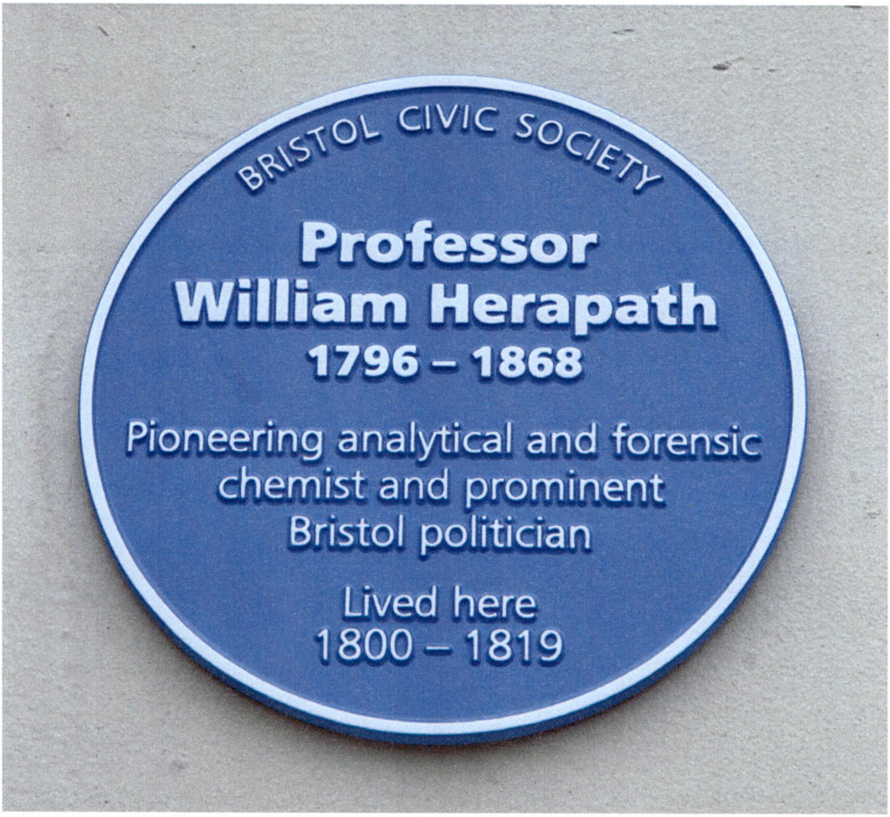

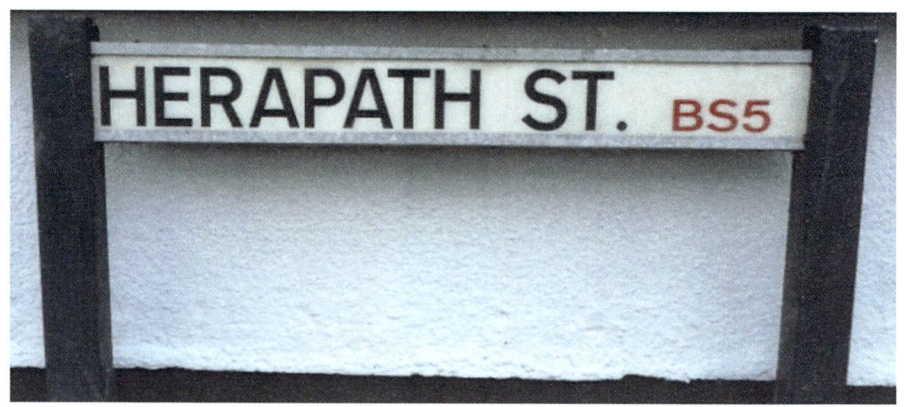

BIBLIOGRAPHY

1] Vincent B. and Holland R., Chemistry in Bristol into the Early 20th Century, ALHA books no 18, Bristol, 2014.

2] Stock J.E., Memoirs of the Life of Thomas Beddoes, MD, John Murray, London, 1811.

3] Stansfield D.A., Thomas Beddoes, MD, 1760-1808, Chemist, Physician, Democrat, Reidel, Dordrecht, 1984.

4] Neve M., Beddoes, Thomas (1760-1808), Oxford Dictionary of National Biography, Oxford University Press, 2004.

5] Jay M., The Atmosphere of Heaven: The Unnatural Experiments of Dr Beddoes and His Sons of Genius, Yale University Press, 2009.

6] Watson K.D., Herapath, William (1796–1868), Oxford Dictionary of National Biography, Oxford University Press, 2004.

7] Vincent B., The Herapaths of Bristol: a Medical and Scientific Dynasty, ALHA books no 21, Bristol, 2016.

A History of Caesarean Birth

by Thomas F. Baskett

BOOK REVIEW BY PAUL GODDARD

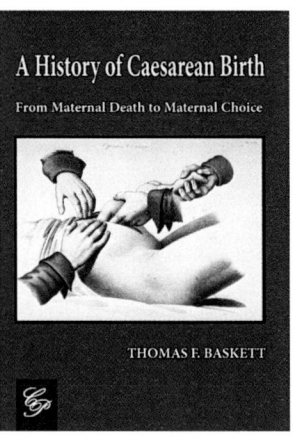

Professor Baskett presented the history of Caesarean Birth to the Bristol Medico-Historical Society on 24th April 2017 and then wrote up his research as an excellent book of the same title. Caesarean birth is the stuff of legend. The god of medicine, Aesculapius, is said to have been delivered by an abdominal incision, Buddha similarly. Julius Caesar, Robert II of Scotland, Edward VI of England.... the list continues but most are stated as being apocryphal. Post-mortem caesarean delivery has a more convincing history and when the book gets into the examples of self performed caesarean section it becomes addictive reading. Until the late nineteenth century operating a c. section on yourself was safer than letting the surgeons get at you! In fact delivery by being gored by a bull was safer than submitting to the surgeons. For example a mother of three children in Mexico in 1830 was gored by a bull whilst milking a cow. The baby boy was immediately expelled... *"When her distressed daughters came to her assistance she instructed them to get brandy, needle and thread. Whereupon she washed the wound with the brandy, stitched the abdominal wound and walked into the house."* The child survived and she went on to have three more successful pregancies and deliveries. The book continues with similarly interesting anecdotes but also wise words about the importance of caesarean birth in reducing infant and maternal mortality.

Published by Clinical Press ISBN 978-1-85457-065-9 £19.00

Agatha Christie, Queen of Crime
and her deadly dispensary of poison
Presented to the Bristol Medico-Historical Society 16th October 2017

JANET SELLICK
email: janetsellick@gmail.com

"Surrounded by poisons I suppose it was natural I should use poison as the murderer's weapon in my very first book," said Agatha Christie about the start of her remarkable career. To lighten the dark subject of murder and poison we'll look at how her beloved Devon inspired her writing. Her own life was as dramatic and eventful as her fiction. We'll discover people, places and plants that inspired her to become the most popular crime writer of all time. We'll look back at the tradition of crime writing of her time and also consider her legacy both local and global.

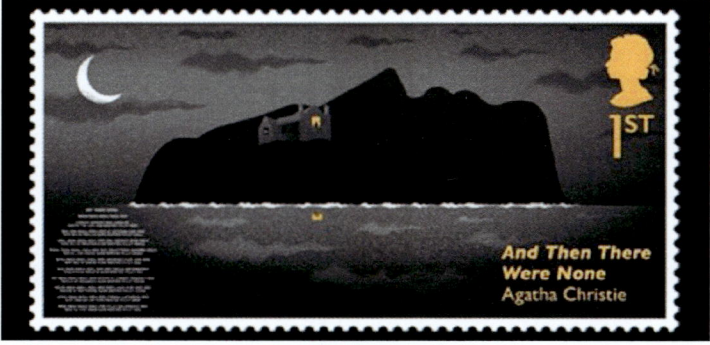

Figure 1
Burgh Island Stamp

In the best Agatha Christie tradition we start with a mystery. This Royal Mail postage stamp of Burgh Island was launched in 2016 to celebrate the centenary of Agatha Christie writing her first novel *"The Mysterious Affair at Styles"*. Jim Sutherland, one of the stamp designers, wanted them to reflect Christie's consummate skill in confusing her readers.

Burgh Island was the inspiration for Agatha's all-time best seller *"And Then There Were None"* written in 1939. The island as shown is also a man's profile looking up to the sky; the little yellow hotel light is his eye. This conjures up the sinister presence of the murderer who invites guests to stay, strands them on the island only to kill them off one by one, sometimes violently, sometimes discreetly by poison.

By the time she died in 1976, she was the world's best selling crime writer. According to the Guinness Book of Records this is still true. Only outsold by the Bible and Shakespeare she wrote over a hundred books and plays in a career spanning more than fifty years. Sales of her works are four million annually. Two billion copies have been sold worldwide, translated into 130 languages.

In 1968 she was made Dame Commander of the Order of the British Empire. She was unpretentious and modest, insisting she wanted her books to just entertain; a shy person, she shunned publicity. She was an expert in archaeology and photography. She read and spoke excellent French.

In 1938 she purchased Greenway, her beloved holiday home on the river Dart in Devon. She became a passionate plants woman. She had a very fine singing voice and was an accomplished pianist. She volunteered to nurse in Torquay Hospital during the first World War and was swiftly promoted to the hospital dispensary.

"The Mysterious Affair at Styles" written in 1916 had a dramatic description of the symptoms of death by strychnine poisoning. It was praised for its accuracy by the *"Pharmaceutical Journal and Pharmacist."* A review that she cherished all her life. A hundred years later her use of science has been put under scrutiny again, this time by Professor of Toxicology Kathryn Harkup in her erudite and fascinating book *"A is for Arsenic"*. Harkup's explanations of how the various poisons attack the body makes beautiful science and scary reading.

Professor Harkup concludes that Christie's science was almost without exception, correct. She writes: *"Throughout her writing career Christie kept up to date with the safe and dangerous use of drugs. She collected articles about real live murder cases. Her notes showed she studied some of the more lurid murderers such as Crippen."*

Christie's detailed descriptions of Thallium poisoning in *"The Pale Horse"* in 1961 were used by pathologists who were examining one of the victims killed by the real life serial killer Graham Young in 1962.

Her arsenal of poisons contains Arsenic, Belladonna, Curare Digitalis, Eserine, Hemlock, Monkshood, Nicotine, Opium, Phosphorus, Ricin, Strychnine and Veronal. *"A deadly dispensary"* indeed, as Professor Harkup termed it..

Let's start with the common foxglove. In *"Appointment with Death"*, set on an archeological dig in Petra, the murderer was fortunate to be travelling with a doctor who had digitalis in his bag to treat the victim who was already suffering from a heart complaint. An extra dose proved lethal. This went unnoticed by all except Poirot.

Nearly all Christie's potent plants can be seen in Torre Abbey in Torquay. The head gardener Ali Marshal has created a beautiful potent plant garden inspired by Christie's use of poisons, all part of Christie's legacy in Devon.

Professor Harkup examines her use of arsenic, ricin and phosphorus.

Arsenic, *"The King of poison and poison of Kings"* only killed eight out of the more than 300 characters dispatched by Christie. It was already known in the time of Cleopatra. When she decided to kill herself it is said she tried various poisons on her slaves and watched the results. Arsenic was too unpleasant for Cleo, so she chose the asp. Arsenic was often a poisoner's first choice as it has no taste. Symptoms of arsenic poisoning resemble food poisoning and dysentery. Arsenic was also the centre of great speculation about the death of Napoleon Bonaparte in 1821.

He suffered from severe stomach aches, and French and British accused the other of poisoning him. 140 years later analysis of a hair sample showed it had a higher than usual but non-fatal arsenic level. The wallpaper was the culprit, arsenic gas had been produced by the paste. He had also been given a tonic containing potassium arsenite.

In *"Murder is Easy"* victims are drowned, pushed under a bus, into a canal, out of a window and hit over the head, and of course, poisoned. Those victims had all complained to the doctor of severe recurrent stomach pains. In the end the killer confesses to having killed the unfortunate Mrs Horton by dissolving arsenic trioxide in a hot cup of tea.

Christie sought ever more devious and ingenious ways for her murderers to administer and conceal their choice of poison.

In *"The House of Lurking Death"* an extract from the castor oil plant, ricin, killed all the victims. There were castor oil plants in the garden. Miss Logan had many pinpricks on her arm. She claimed from a rose bush but that rose bush had no thorns. Miss Logan had been injecting herself with small doses of ricin so that when she offered a plate of ricin enriched fig sandwiches to all her guests she ate a little too. She became ill but survived and therefore was not a suspect. The parlour maid was not supposed to be a victim. She purloined a sandwich in the pantry. Her greed was indeed a deadly sin.

Some critics have said that Christie's use of poisons is often too contrived and unrealistic, but one of the most extraordinary modern assassinations ever took place in London in 1978. The Bulgarian defector George Markov was walking over Waterloo Bridge when a passerby thrust his umbrella at his leg. The tiny capsule later found in his leg was found by Porton Down to have contained the fatal dose: Ricin.

In her first novel *"The Mysterious Affair at Styles"* the Inglethorpe family visit a local pharmacist friend. A bottle of strychnine is on the shelf. All the suspects are there and are able to steal it if they wished. Poirot finds strychnine in a drawer, purchased to put down a dog, as one could do in those days. It was also sold as pesticide. He finds strychnine in the tonic beside the victim's bed. In 1916 none of this was in itself unduly suspicious.

In *"The Dumb Witness"* the murderer chooses phosphorus as his murder weapon. Miss Arundell was taking liver pills in the form of gelatin capsules. It was easy for the murderer to empty the capsules and refill them with 100 mg of phosphorus. In those days phosphorus was easy to obtain as a rat poison.

*

A break from murder now to explore what else inspired her. Born September 15, 1890 in Torquay she was the youngest of Frederick and Clara Miller's three children. She was schooled in her father's extensive library at her beloved home Ashfield.

As a tourist guide with foreign groups I have seen first hand how Agatha's Christie's works are held in such high esteem abroad. Many teachers use her works to teach English conversation. Agatha Christie brings thousands of visitors to Devon. It often seems like a pilgrimage.

There is even a walk called the Agatha Christie Mile. A favourite spot on this walk is Beacon Cove. Agatha almost drowned here as a child. Later in her books she does not flinch from death by drowning but only uses it nine times.

When Christie was eleven her father died. His fortune in America was failing. Life at Ashfield had to be less lavish. Her father's death made her realise the necessity of money. Desire for money was to become a recurring motive for resorting to poison again! At this stage in her life though she was a popular young woman mixing with the wealthiest families in Torquay, visiting their grand houses. Many similar houses were to appear in her books.

Agatha had also been a guest on Burgh Island. The visit inspired her to write her best selling book of all time, published in 1939, *"Then There Were None"*. With a hundred million copies sold to date it is now ranked the seventh best selling book of all time. She made a bet that no reader would be able to guess who successfully "bumped off" the ten victims. Burgh Island was also the inspiration for *"Evil under the Sun"*.

*

In 1914 Agatha and Archie were madly in love and at Christmas, she married the impetuous young flying officer in Saint Nicholas church partly visible now in Clifton College. Down in Torquay Agatha's mother had grave misgivings. They enjoyed one night's honeymoon in the elegant Grand Hotel in Torquay. Archie returned to the battlefields of Belgium the very next day. While he was away Agatha started her life long affair with poisons. She was also trying to create her own detective. She was a huge admirer of Sherlock Holmes but wanted her detective to be totally different to him.

The sad groups of Belgian refugees strolling around in Torquay provided her with the very man. She realised that among them must be doctors, nurses, teachers, policemen and why not… a private detective?

So her detective would be foreign, with a pronounced foreign accent in sharp contrast to the quintessentially English Sherlock. He was tall and slim. Hers would be short and portly. The name would be slightly humorous. Poirot sounds like the French for the vegetable leek. With his fastidiously waxed moustaches he was hardly Hercules. Hercule Poirot was born.

While studying for her Apothecary exams she met a pharmacist in Torquay who inspired her murder plots with unusual poisons. She refers to the chemist as Mr. P. A disturbing character. He told her how he felt powerful by carrying a solid piece of curare, another deadly poison, around in his pocket. This may well have been the trigger for her interest in the more esoteric poisons.

In the final Poirot book *"Curtain"*, Hastings' daughter is in love with a slightly obsessive scientist researching the Calabar bean. The scientist's wife is murdered. Hastings even believes his daughter could be suspect. A baffling plot finishes off Poirot. The local name for the bean was eséré. The same compound is also known as esserine and is used in the ophthalmic industry. Christie used it in *"The Crooked House"* to kill off a victim who was given his eye drops to drink.

In *"The Pale Horse"* the murderer uses thallium, a soft grey metal which is used in photography. A group of people interested in the occult meet in the Pale Horse pub. There is of course a murderer in their midst.

*

In 1926 an event equally baffling and worthy of any of her own Whodunnits brought her international fame. Her disappearance on December 3rd caused the police to suspect her husband Archie Christie had murdered her. He was having an affair with a brunette called Nancy Neele. Agatha Christie's car had been found abandoned in an isolated spot in Surrey.

An enormous manhunt was launched with over 15,000 volunteers. Ten days later she was found in a hotel in Harrogate in Yorkshire. A statement was released saying she had suffered an attack of amnesia. She refused to ever speak of the incident again. This unexplained event may well have inspired several modern writers. *"Gone Girl"* by Gillian Flynn for example.

It definitely inspired Andrew Wilson to write *"A Talent for Murder"*. Published in May 2017 he takes her disappearance and creates a baffling scenario to explain her bizarre behaviour.

She wrote in that time often called the Golden Age of British detective fiction: 1920 -1945: The era of the locked room, the country house murder, the snow covered lawn with no footprints.

Ingenuity reached new heights – the poison smeared postage stamp and the icicle dagger soon to melt into thin air. In 1944 a board game called Murder was invented to help pass the time in bombshelters. Waddingtons snapped it up and renamed it *"Cluedo"*.

By the outbreak of War Agatha Christie was a household name. Her books were the must-have reading material in the underground. They were soothing! Readers waited anxiously for her next book. She was dubbed the Queen of Crime, the Duchess of Death. In *"Lord Edgware Dies"* he is stabbed by a dagger in the library in true Colonel Mustard tradition. Some critics have called Christie formulaic, with her characters pushed around a Cluedo board. Not always.

The *"Murder of Roger Ackroyd"* written in 1926 caused a huge storm of critical accusations that Christie had cheated her readers. Despite this, it is still one of her best sellers. On a Radio 4 Book Club discussion it was held up as an example of the best crime fiction ever.

If Christie's style is formulaic, it's a winning formula with the enduring power of Miss Marple and Poirot. He was created in her very first book in 1916. Readers had to wait till 1932 for Miss Marple. She never lets them meet. Miss Marple has a very firm fan base who relish her ruthless pursuit of truth.

*

The public has however always clamoured for Poirot. *"A Christie for Christmas"* was the cry. She, however, wanted to dispatch Poirot. She wrote *"Curtain" i*n 1940. Her publishers refused to let her kill him. She kept the book hidden for thirty-five years. It was eventually published in 1975 just four months before she died.

Poirot's last case caused a sensation: the first ever Obituary to a fictional detective was published in the New York Times on August 6th 1975: *"Hercule Poirot, a Belgian detective who became internationally famous, has died in England. His age was unknown".*

Of course he lives on. Through TV, radio, stage and films both Poirot and Miss Marple have gained new fans. The ITV productions of Poirot with David Suchet are as popular in Bucharest as Bristol.

*

It seems we have an insatiable appetite for crime fiction. Some of us delight in a smorgasbord of violence in the Scandi noirs or the gentler scenes with Morse morphing into Lewis, and of course Poirot where lurid descriptions of torture and agonizing deaths are rare. For the accused and victims their agony is the paranoia when they realize a murderer is often under the same roof. Why do we enjoy this so?

Amanda Ellison, a scientist in the cognitive neuroscience research unit at Durham University, has stated, *"Well written crime dramas, with complex plots and red herrings provide the sort of stimulation the brain craves."*

All Christie fans love the final pages of the mysteries when the murderer is revealed. Clues abound, often unnoticed in conversation. A body sprawled on the beach is not necessarily a corpse. Mistrust the friend offering you a friendly nightcap. It could be laced with morphine or worse. Above all, never trust the family doctor and don't drop your guard at a cocktail party. The unfortunate Reverend Babbington, dropped his when he took a second slurp of a bitter tasting cocktail. In *"Three Act Tragedy"* that unpleasant taste was not Campari but nicotine. Two minutes later he was dead, sprawled on the floor.

*

Agatha wrote eighty-three murder mysteries, over one hundred short stories and eighteen plays. *"She was at home on the stage as much as on the page"* writes John Curran in *"Agatha Christie's Secret Notebooks".* Her most famous play is *"The Mousetrap",* the longest running play in theatre history. It has now run for over sixty-five years! Her non-fiction work *"Come Tell Me How You Live"* describes her life in the Middle East, on archeological digs with her second husband, Max Mallowan. Agatha took countless photos of objects on site, developing the photos in very primitive lab conditions in the desert. She wrote *"Death in Mesopotamia"* and *"They Came to Baghdad"* in situ. She even started her autobiography in Nimrud. Nothing could stop her writing.

In Max she found her soul mate. A journalist, Beverley Nichols, attributed these words to Agatha: *"The good thing marrying an archaeologist is, the older you get, the more interested in you he is"*. Her legacy in Devon is Greenway: her hideaway, where she could be herself and read her latest mystery to the family. I was at Greenway once when after dinner, Matthew Pritchard, Christie's grandson, read the opening chapter of *"Ordeal by Innocence"*. Matthew's voice drew us into the description of a night full of foreboding.   We all sensed the menacing gloom near the river as a stranger catches the ferry. The steady plash of the oars brings him nearer to an ordeal he dreads. Greenway Quay and the ferry were vividly described. I won't continue as spoilers are taboo. Matthew's reading changed my view profoundly about his grandmother's works. It was the start of seeing her as more than a clever plotter of Who Dunnits imbued with dreadful deaths and poisons. The insight into the lonely traveller's mind was worthy of a dark moody psychological thriller.

In *"Deadman's Folly"* Greenway is again used as the location. Greenway is visible too in *"Five Little Pigs"*. There the victim is poisoned with hemlock, the symptoms similar to those of Socrates' harrowing death.

*

Poison so often adds dramatic interest and shock to the plot, but poison is only the WHAT that kills the victim. The page turner is the HOW it is planned and secretly administered. Sleuths, sometimes Poirot, sometimes Miss Marple, sometimes the readers succeed in uncovering the WHO in Whodunnit.

It has been said that once the villain is identified a sort of status quo is restored or is it? Is it a true happy ending? As Sarah Phelps of the BBC says, *"Status, faith and relationships are revealed as based on deceit and lies."* However lighthearted and cosy some critics find her works, murder is a dark gruesome thing. Families are shattered. Sarah Phelps is presently adapting three Christie works. New to Agatha Christie she was shocked by the savagery in *"Then There Were None"*. She was determined to emulate the simmering menace of the *"ruthless, remorseless murderer who gives the victims no chance to plead. Nowhere to hide."* Aiden Turner of Poldark starred in her production. The paranoia felt by the victims stranded on the island sheds any cosy image of Christie's writing. The Times in May 2017 ran an article entitled *"How Christie got Cool"*.

*

Her fan base has widened with the digital age. We can get her on our Kindle or download an app. We can enjoy her in the cinema and of course on TV.

On the big screen is Kenneth Branagh's new exciting film of *"Murder on the Orient Express"*. The novel written in 1934 is rated second favourite by fans. It notched up three million sales in 1974 alone, the year it was made into a film with Albert Finney as Poirot.

This year's version has Branagh as Poirot. The palpable suspense is within the claustrophobic train among the travellers all under suspicion of murder. It is hoped to bring in new fans to the Christie brand while maintaining the Christie "must have": a surprise twist revealed by Poirot. Among the cast are Judy Dench and Derek Jacobi along with Hollywood's Johnny Depp, Penelope Cruz and Michelle Pfeiffer.

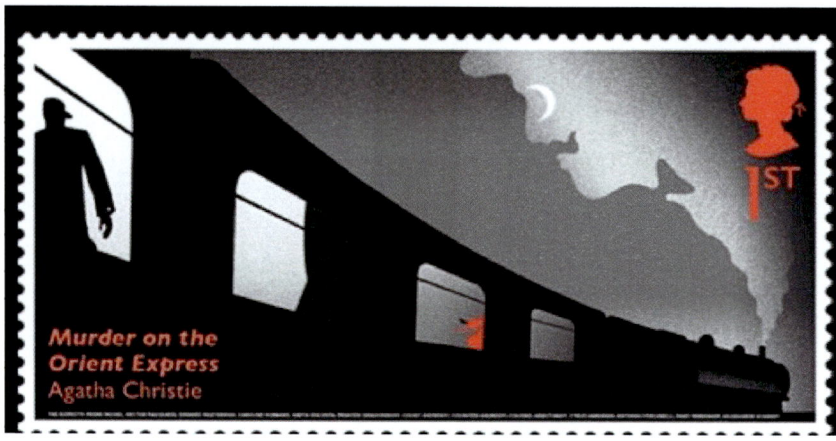

Figure 2 The Orient Express Stamp

Note the figure in red fleeing along the corridor. A vital clue. Of course there's a hidden treasure in this image. Just stare at the smoke. Can you see a man's profile hidden in it? If not, start at the top with the brim of his hat. Go down to the moon, his monocle. Below that is his moustache and finally on down to his bow tie.

Ladies and Gentlemen I leave you with… Hercule Poirot.

Richard Smith
Surgeon, Poet and Collector

MIKE WHITFIELD

Presented at the Bristol Medico-Historical Society meeting on 19.3.2018

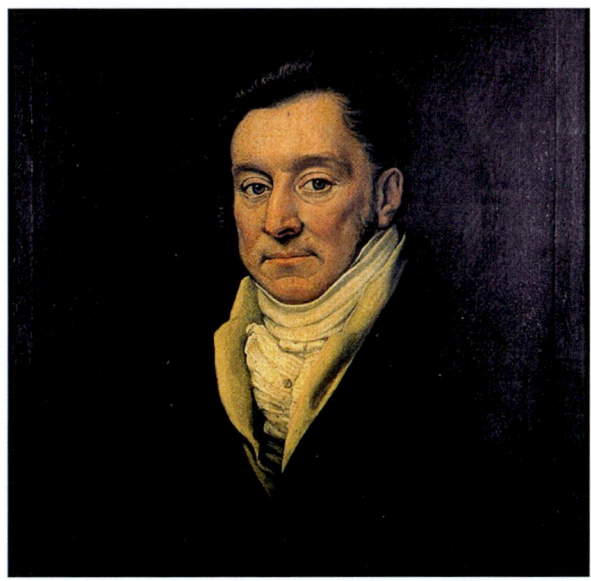

Richard Smith

Richard Smith lived at the beginning of the nineteenth century – it was an exciting time in Bristol. The war with France had ended. There were at least two major riots in the city. The Luddites were destroying agricultural machinery in the fields. Change in Britain was being encouraged by the French revolution and the poets Southey and Coleridge were living next door to Smith in College Green.

It was 1835 and there was a report in The Lancet about an operation on an aneurysm of the external iliac artery that had been performed by Smith who was 63 years old. The report had been written anonymously, as was the custom in that 10 year old radical medical journal. The writer was obviously a surgeon himself and who had said that he asked for permission to see the operation as he was visiting the city.

The Bristol Infirmary is a well-appointed and well-regulated establishment. It possesses a good library, a fine museum and able professional officers, and must afford to students an admirable field for obtaining medical and surgical knowledge.

The operation room is spacious, light and well ventilated. The gallery is carried three parts round, there is plenty of accommodation and the discipline is excellent. None but the officers of the house and the pupils of the operating surgeon are ever permitted to occupy the area of the floor, so there is no bustle, or calling out of "heads". In fact, the spectators can witness what is going on in a comfortable and satisfactory manner.

We waited around impatiently, almost an hour, when Mr Richard Smith, the senior surgeon, came into the room and said "Gentlemen, I am sorry to inform you that I cannot persuade the man to subject to the operation, although he had distinctly consented to it; but if I can hereafter alter his resolution, I shall be happy to see you again." We departed much disappointed. A week elapsed, and on the 21st we again assembled. In a few minutes the patient was brought in, seemingly care-worn and woe-begone. He was aged about 40, and dated his malady to a kick from a rioter, when the prison was burned in October 1831, he being a turnkey.

The operator drew his scalpel at one sweep through the integuments in a somewhat semilunar direction, making a wound about five inches long, and ending at the upper edge of the tumour. Laying aside his knife, the way was cleared with both hands down to the psoas muscle, and the operator began to search the cavity. One of the surgeons who was near, asked "Do you feel the artery?"

"Yes, distinctly, and it is a good deal bound down, but I think I shall soon be able to detach it with my finger and thumb." Presently

Mr Smith said, "Now I have the artery over my finger." "is it quite free?" "Yes, there is nothing but the artery; I am quite sure of it; favour me with the blunt needle with the ligature". The instrument broke from the handle, another was substituted, and the needle was passed very readily under the vessel. A surgeon pulled up the ligature with a dissecting forceps, and the needle was then withdrawn. The silk was now under the artery. The operator drew up the ends, so as to bring the sides of the artery in contact. "Gentlemen, will you satisfy yourselves that the circulation is commanded? Three or four hands in succession were laid upon the tumour. "Yes, the pulsation is gone - it is all right - the sooner you tie the better". The ligature was then tightened and the operation finished. The integuments were drawn together with adhesive plaster, a strip of lint and a bandage was applied, and the patient was carried out. The operation occupied under ten minutes, and there was not a tablespoon of blood spilled from first to last. After the first incision, the patient appeared scarcely to suffer at all. The operation gave universal satisfaction. It was performed with the utmost coolness, and in a surgeon-like manner. I have seen Sir Astley Cooper perform the operation twice and I have seen three other hospital surgeons perform it in London, but this operation, in my judgement, might dispute the palm with any of them, The utmost attention also was evinced by the other four surgeons, Mesrs Hetling, Lowe, Daniel and Nat Smith, and the duties of Mr Morgan, the house-surgeon, were performed with promptness.

Five days have now elapsed, and I understand that the man has had not one unpleasant symptom; he has slept well; there has been no tension of the abdomen; the wound exhibits a mere line, the tumour sinks, and the limb is of a comfortable temperature. The case is the second of the kind which has occurred in the house. Mr Smith has been surgeon for nearly forty years.*

The *Lancet* publication clearly stimulated Smith to write a letter to the editor describing the state of his patient two months later:

> To inform you that Ricketts had not one unpleasant symptom from the moment when he was carried to bed to the present time. His gloomy despair soon left him, and was succeeded by a confident and cheering view. In about a week the wound was entirely closed, with the exception only of the part situated in the course of the ligature. From this period there was discharged during each day about an ounce of good pus. On the 30th day after the operation the ligature was found coiled up in the dressing and shortly after the man walked home without any difficulty.

Smith had a particular interest in bladder stones, and he studied the outcome of lithotomy operations, writing about frequency of such operations in Bristol and throughout England and their prevalence and mortality rates.

Surgery in the early nineteenth century

The four surgeons in the Infirmary worked together much more than they do today: In the year 1839 there were 74 meetings (of the surgeons) held in the consulting room when the cases of 137 patients were brought seriatim under their notice, minutely examined and a record immediately entered of the decisions, whether for operation or a plan of treatment: at these meetings, in four-fifths of the instances, from four to five of the surgeons were present, indeed it was only in about four or five cases of sudden casualties that as few as three were present.

Henry Alford, who spent a year as Smith's pupil, became a surgeon himself and wrote an article in 1890 about his experience as a medical student in Bristol in 1822. He wrote:

Smith was a good surgeon for those days; rather careless in the treatment of his patients, whether in the wards or in the operating theatre. He was a bold, steady operator, but rather rough and reckless; and not very mindful of the feelings or state of his patient. He was very popular with the pupils and his colleagues, and I think,

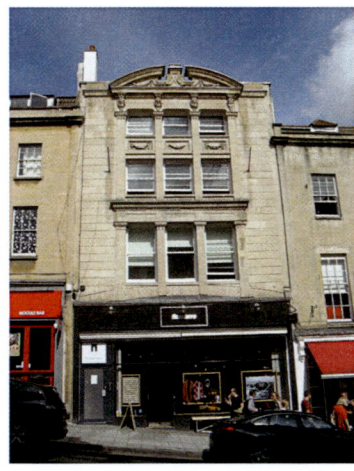

Smith's Park Street House

rather a favourite with the Infirmary patients. He was in the habit of seeing patients in his own house (see above) of a morning, mostly young men, and dispensing for them in a very rough way from his own surgery. One of his pupils attended there for an hour or two every morning, to show the patients into Mr Smith's consulting-room; they generally came by a back door opening into Park Row. Mr Smith lived in Park Street, and to dispense the medicines prescribed, usually verbally, and mostly limited to powders, pills, or ointment, put up in a very rough and ready style.

Early professional experience

In 1795, Richard completed his training as a surgeon and on the front door of his mother's house in College Street he advertised himself as Richard Smith, Surgeon and on the back door in Lamb Street, he was Richard Smith, Surgeon and Apothecary. He was appointed surgeon at the Infirmary aged 24 in 1796

With Francis Bowles, he was involved with two series of anatomical lectures, the first in 1797. These were instigated by Dr Thomas Beddoes as part of his initiative in preventive medicine

The Collector

Smith was a great collector, the most important of his collections are his fourteen enormous scrapbooks about medical life in and around Bristol. He also produced three scrapbooks about theatre memorabilia including details of the Jacob's Well theatre and the Theatre Royal.

He and his father were largely responsible for creating the Infirmary museum, which at one time was considered second to the Hunterian museum in London and unfortunately is now destroyed.

He also left a collection of receipts from February 1829 to October 1830. These give a good indication of some of his household expenses during those two years. For example, from January 13 1830 to March 5 there is a receipt for 10 cwt of coal every 2 weeks until 5 March at 18 shillings a time. He paid 25 shillings for a half year's supply of gas from the Bristol Gas-light Company. On 29 May he paid £2 for a half-year's Poor Rate and on 2 June 1829 £1 1s 9d for a half year's taxes (10s 6d windows and 11s 3d house) to the Out-Parish of St Philip & Jacob. There was a *'composition Rate on the Highways'* of £5 7s 6d.

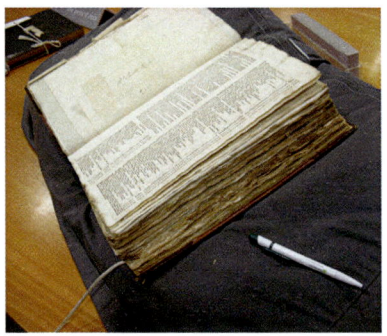

Biographical memoir

The most frequent receipts, though, were for alcohol. He seems to have purchased a barrel of beer containing 54 gallons at least once a fortnight from a wide variety of breweries. He also bought a hundred clay pipes.

The Poet and writer

From 1804 until 1820 Smith became one of the proprietors of the Bristol Mirror, a local weekly newspaper and occasionally would write for this, usually anonymously. In 1806, under the pseudonym Simpkin he wrote a poem about the local surgeons and one verse was about himself:

> *There is R.S. Who reads and rolls on in his gig,*
> *With a coachman beside him as fat as a pig;*
> *Whilst Traveller and Spot, two dogs of a kind,*
> *Like a couple of footmen keep trotting behind.*
> *Only kick up a row. And he's sure to be nibbling,*
> *Being never so happy as when he's a scribbling.*

> *But you'll not be surprised, I'm quite sure, on this score,*
> *Since 'twas just the same thing with his DADDY of yore.*

Smith was fascinated with murders. He wrote about two historical murders and had first hand contact with at least two murderers. The first of these was John Horwood.

There was a series of letters between Messrs Browne and Watson, solicitors to the parents of John Horwood and Richard Smith in the local newspaper, in which they request that the dissection does not take place, to *"spare the distress of Horwood's parents"* and Smith replies:

The father and brother of the unfortunate malefactor have probably informed you, that I have had with them, at my house, this morning, a most painful interview; and, certainly, if I had permitted my feelings to have assumed the mastery over my sense of duty in this miserable affair, the tears of so respectable old man would, as far as I was personally concerned, have prevailed, and forced me to yield to his solicitations.

The next day Smith described how he dissected the body in front of an invited audience of 80 people and completed the dissection on the following day. Horwood's skin was tanned and prepared as the covering of a book that contains the phrenograph of John Horwood (an example of the pseudo-science of that day which purported to show the character of Horwood) and other papers relating to the case. The book was embossed with the words Cutis vera Johannis Horwood and still resides in the Bristol museum.

Smith's skill in describing Mrs Burdock, another murderer, and her reaction to her trial is outstanding.:

Whilst she was at the bar she ate sandwiches and drank a glass of beer, which she carried to her mouth with the utmost steadiness and indifference. After condemnation, having descended from the pen into the room below, she burst out into a furious rage, swore and blasphemed, cursed the recorder and the counsel both pro and con, and damned her advocates for not seizing the favourable points in her case.

Sir John Dinely's murder was described in three sections in weekly editions of the Bristol Mirror and was in the following form illustrated with the following excerpts:

That is a murderer's gibbet! Yes, in chains
there hung Mahoney's body – his remains
Have long since disappeared – a savoury dish
once for the ravenous gulls and Portishead fish.
Which they did breakfast, dine and sup
Until the murderer was eaten up.

The third part of 'The Fratricide' ends with a detailed description of Captain Dinely's dissection in the Infirmary:

In oilcased sleeves the Surgeons now begin
To divide "The Integuments", that is, the skin
And membranes cellular, and now so nice
The incision crucial's made, and in a trice
The hundreds gaping on begin to see
Into the chest and lower cavity.....

Mrs Runscombe and her maid were murdered in 1764. Smith described the large rewards that were offered and the various suspects that were investigated, but no one was ever prosecuted for this terrible murder. He concluded: *Such are the particulars of a murder perpetrated in open day, whilst the people in numbers were passing and repassing the door just behind which were bodies, and that within a few yards of the Cathedral, and during Divine service: and yet, from that moment even to this, the whole matter was and is involved in total darkness, and so will now probably remain to the Day of Judgement.*

Alford described Smith and his family:

He was a big burly man with a round florid face, large whiskers, a hearty, jovial manner and rather loud, brusque voice. He was a boon companion in society, and a welcome guest at public and private dinners, He could tell a good story or anecdote, and, I believe, sing a comic song, His tales were often professional and neither those nor some of his jokes or songs were quite suitable for the ears of ladies, or clergymen, or non-professional gentlemen. But in those days a good deal of coarseness in language was not only tolerated, but looked for and enjoyed at public gatherings.

His brother Henry's early adult life was complicated by mortally wounding a man in a duel in 1809.

Alford continued: *His wife was well known and highly esteemed in Bristol as a very benevolent lady, and an active, earnest member of the Evangelical Church party, with whom she was reported to have kept up a good deal of visiting at her own house. But it was understood that her husband was never, or very rarely, present at these parties. I believe they lived very amicably in the same house, but had each their different friends and pursuits. I have an idea that Mrs Smith had a private carriage for herself.*

Smith's other interests included:
- Charity Work
- Local councillor from 1835
- Glee Club
- Membership and office holder in Freemasonry
- Membership and office holder in the Bristol Institute
- Theatre buff

Smith died of a stroke on January 24 1843 and his funeral was witnessed by a large proportion of the population of Bristol as the procession made its way from his house in Park Street to Temple church. The streets were lined with spectators and scarcely a window was unoccupied. The pall was borne by all of the physicians and surgeons of the Infirmary.

****

Further details about the life of Richard Smith are contained in his biography: *Richard Smith: Bristol Surgeon and Medical Collector* 1772-1843 by Michael Whitfield ALHA Books No.26

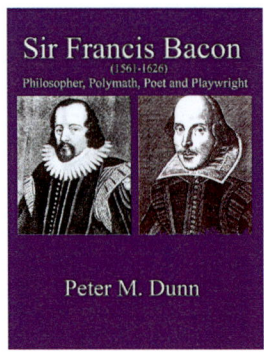

Sir Francis Bacon
BY PETER M DUNN
Monday 11th December 2017

Professor Dunn presented a lecture on the life of Sir Francis Bacon and put this together as a short book that is a companion to the proceedings of the society. ISBN 9781854570956 £10.00

The Evolution of Pre-hospital Emergency Care

BY JOHN GEDDES, RONALD STEWART AND THOMAS BASKETT

Reviewed by Paul R Goddard

Professor Tom Baskett was kind enough to give another presentation to the society on 30th April 2018, just over a year after his talk on Caesarean Birth. This was on *Frank Pantridge and the Evolution of Pre-hospital Emergency Care* and was also put together as a book. The talk and the book covered the early development of mobile coronary care within the context of major societal and scientific changes.

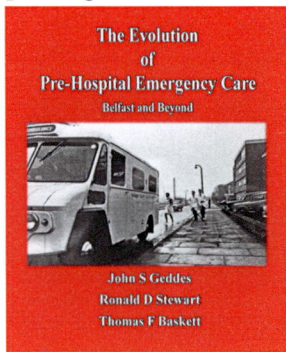

The success of the Belfast Cardiac Ambulance stimulated the development of broader pre-hospital emergency services. The importance of Frank Pantridge in this progress cannot be over-estimated.
ISBN 978-1-85457-093-2 £20.00

The Story of the Hotwell at Bristol

PAUL G N MAIN MA MB BCHIR, FRCGP, FHEA
Retired GP and Honorary Senior Lecturer, School of Social and Community Medicine,
University of Bristol

Presented to the Bristol Medico-Historical Society 16th October 2018

Two years ago I attended a course of lectures in London on the History of Medicine organised by the Worshipful Society of Apothecaries. It was suggested that the participants might like to do some research using primary sources and write a dissertation. Some of the lectures were given by medical doctors and some by professional historians. One historian said that doctors tended to be more interested in famous doctors and historians were more interested in patients [1].

So I decided to research the patients who attended the Hotwell as it was just a stone's throw from where I live. Regarding the Hotwell patients my initial idea was to look at:

1. Who were they?
2. Where did they come from?
3. What was their age, gender, class, occupation?
4. What illnesses did they have?
5. What treatment did they have?
6. Who provided that treatment: apothecaries, barber-surgeons or physicians?
7. What were the outcomes?

Using primary sources proved to be difficult as there were no records as you would find in a hospital or dispensary. There were a number of sequential books written by various doctors each one referring back to earlier ones and adding their own thoughts, opinions and sometimes analysis of the water.

The main authors were Dr Tobias Venner of Bath (1620), Dr Thomas Johnson (1634), Dr Thomas Guidot of Bath (1691), Dr John Underhill of Bristol (1703), Dr Benjamin Allen (1706), Dr

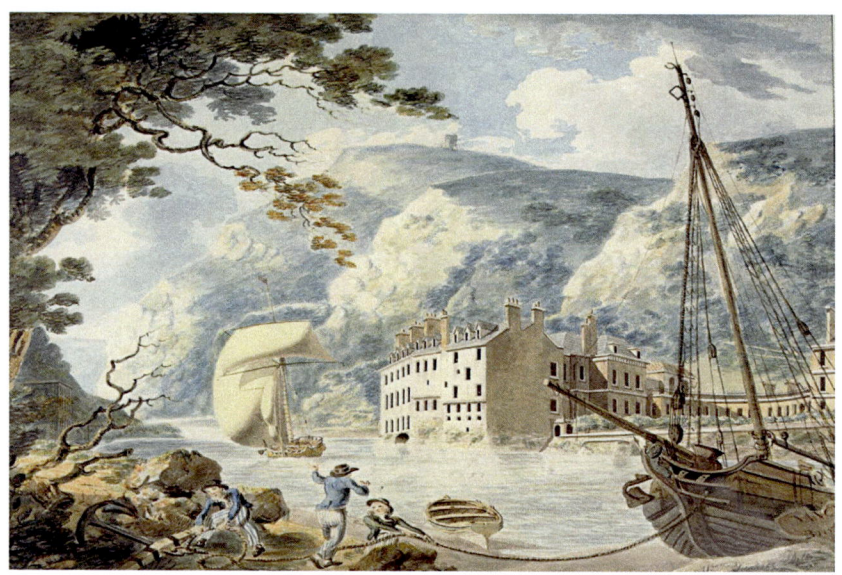
*'The Rising Squall: Avon Gorge and the Bristol Hotwell'
by JMW Turner age 16, 1792*

George Randolph of Bristol (1750), Dr John Rutty (1757), Dr A Sutherland of Bath (1758), Dr Diederick Linden (1759), Dr Andrew Carrick of Clifton (1789), Dr John Nott of Hotwells (1973)[2].

The most useful of these was written by Dr John Underhill of Bristol, who, practising in College Green, published in 1703 a collection of 34 cases consisting of children and adults up to the age of 77 [3].

The heyday of the Hotwell at Bristol was mainly during the reign of the Georgian Kings from 1714 -1830. During that period, Bristol was England's second city in terms of population, and particularly wealth, which was largely due to the triangular slave trade.

The Hotwell: location and water

In the Avon Gorge there are several naturally occurring wells and

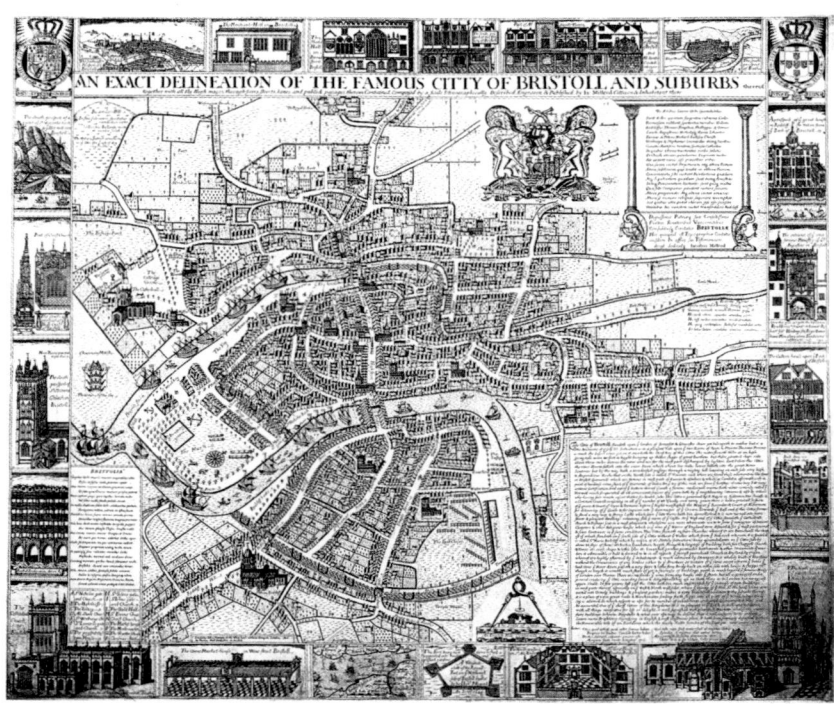

James Millerd's 1673 'An Exact Delineation of the Famous Citty of Bristoll and the suburbs thereof' is the first detailed map of Bristol.

thermal springs. The most famous is known as the Hotwell and it is the warmest 73°-76°F (22.8°-24.4°C). It is thought to have the same source as the Bath Spa waters. Just below St Vincent's Rocks the water bubbled up through rocks and mud, ten feet above low tide mark and twenty-six feet below high water mark. The river Avon has the second highest tidal range in the world after the Bay of Fundy in Nova Scotia.

In 1698, Celia Fiennes, in a travel memoir written for her family, *"Through England on a Side Saddle in the Time of William and Mary"*, described the water *"as warm as new milk and much of that sweetness"*. She went on to say that the water's taste was unlike the sulphurous smell and taste of other British Spas such as Bath, Buxton and Cheltenham.

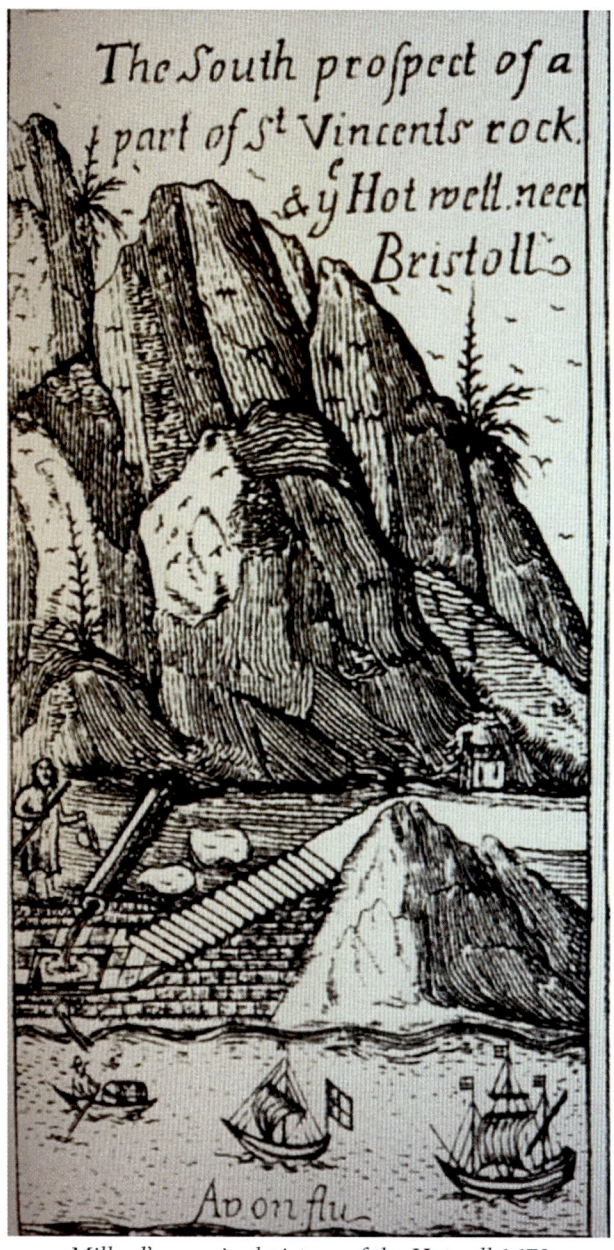

Millerd's marginal picture of the Hotwell 1673

James Millerd produced the first detailed map of Bristol: *'An Exact Delineation of the Famous Citty of Bristoll and the suburbs thereof'* (1673). The map is surrounded by some wonderful marginal pictures of St Mary Redcliffe Church, Bristol Cathedral, Bristol Bridge, St Stephen's Church, the High Cross and the Hotwell. The text on the map gives an interesting description:

'And out of ye bottom thereof issueth a famous warme bath water commonly called ye Hotwell much frequented at all convenient seasons of ye yeare both by ye neighbouring citizens and also by others who liveing farr remote resort thither for health sake.'

Professor William Herapath, a Bristolian, who was a founding fellow of the Chemical Society of London, and also Professor of Chemistry and Toxicology at Bristol Medical School, did a useful analysis of the water in 1854 [4] (see next page).

Hotwell Chronological History

William Wyrecestre (Worcester), an Oxford-educated Bristolian, was an English chronicler, topographer and antiquary. In 1480 he provided the first recorded mention of the Hotwell spring water, saying it was a well known treatment for sailors with scurvy [4].

Early in the seventeenth century, a small brick reservoir was built around the spring, but it was still contaminated at high tide. In 1634, three *'Cavaliers of Norwich'* noted that the waters were used for *"Medicinal purposes and exported to many parts of the world from the port of Bristol"*. In the same year, Thomas Johnson, a London apothecary known as *'The Father of British Field Botany'*, wrote: *"Here from the clefts of the rocks issue forth a spring of warm water pleasant to the taste. It is of some repute and much commended for affections of the kidneys taken inwardly and for old sores applied outwardly"*.

Prof William Herapath's Analysis 1854		Per Imperial gallon
Gas	Formula	Cubic Inches
Carbonic Acid Gas	H_2CO_3	8.76
Nitrogen	N_2	6.56
Solids		Grains
Carbonate of lime	$CaCO_3$	17.7
Sulphate of lime	$CaSO_4$	9.868
Chloride of sodium	NaCl	5.891
Sulphate of soda	Na_2SO_4	3.017
Nitrate of Magnesia	$Mg(NO_3)_2$	2.909
Sulphate of Magnesia	$MgSO_4$	2.267
Chloride of Magnesium	$MgCl_2$	2.18
Carbonate of Magnesia	$MgCO_3$	0.66
Silicia	SiO_2	0.270
Carbonate of Iron	FeCO	0.103
Bitumen		0.15
TOTAL		44.015

Prof William Herapath's Analysis 1854

The Hotwell gained greater respectability and standing when in 1677 Queen Catherine of Braganza, wife of Charles II, visited. In 1694, the first Hotwell House was built, with pumps to raise the spring water up 30ft. It had five storeys, the upper ones being used as lodgings. There was a promenade of trees where

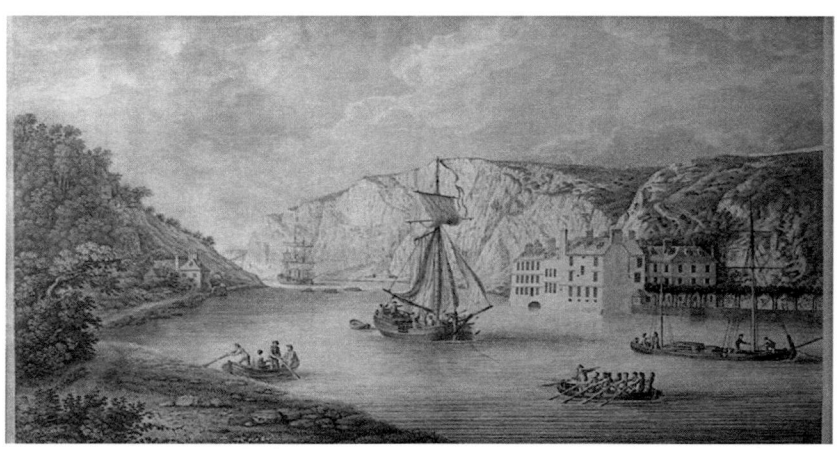

View of Old Hotwell House (1694-1822) & St Vincent's Rock. c1750 from Rownham Ferry (showing Pill hobbler rowing boats)

the visitors could take some exercise and later, in 1786, The Colonnade was built. This contained shops and a lending library run by Ann Yearsley, the Milkmaid Poetess, a protégée of the bluestocking Hannah More, a resident of Clifton.

By the mid-eighteenth century, the Hotwell spring water was *"Not only drunk on the spot at the Pump Room, but every morning cried in the streets like milk"*. The water was sold in the streets every morning, and delivered to any part of the town fresh from the well for six shillings per twelve bottles. It was taken in larger bottles to all parts of England, the Continent, and as far as the West Indies. It retained its properties, unlike Bath Spa water, which therefore wasn't bottled. It was extremely important for the flourishing Bristol glass industry. Back in 1720, Daniel Defoe, in his *'A Tour through the whole island of Great Britain'*, wrote that Bristol was *"The greatest, richest and best port of trade in Great Britain, London only excepted.....there are no less than fifteen glass houses in Bristol, which is more than there are in the city of London. Glass bottles...now used for sending the waters of St Vincent's Rock.... all over the world"* [5]. And by 1739 Alexander Pope counted twenty glass houses, more than

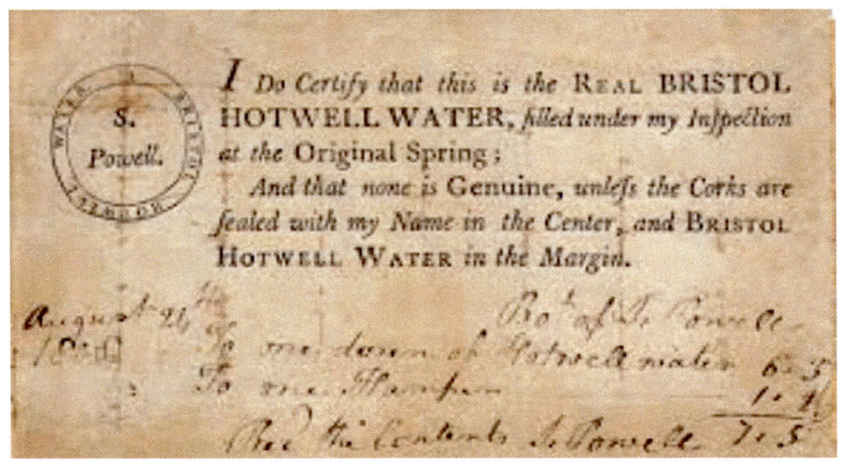

Hotwell bottled water label August 21st 1808.

the church spires of the nineteen parish churches.

'Taking the waters' was now the fashion. Visitors would take a carriage to the Pump Room in the morning, drink the prescribed number of glasses, talk scandal, play cards and listen to the small orchestra. From the Hotwell House the visitors would walk via the tree-lined riverside promenade to the New Vauxhall Pleasure Gardens, where there was more entertainment. In 1795, William Pennington was appointed Master of Ceremonies, a post he held for thirty years. He wore a gold medallion strung on a blue ribbon to emphasise the dignity of his office. He defined the etiquette in the *'Rules of the Hotwell'* which stated: *"That no gentleman appear with a sword or with spurs in these rooms, or on a ball night, in boots. That on all occasions ladies are admitted to these rooms in hats, not excepting the balls given to the Master of the Ceremonies. That the subscription balls will begin as soon as possible after 7 o'clock and concluded at 11, on account of the health of the company"*. He organised public breakfasts, morning concerts, illuminated evening dances, theatre, cards and many other entertainments.

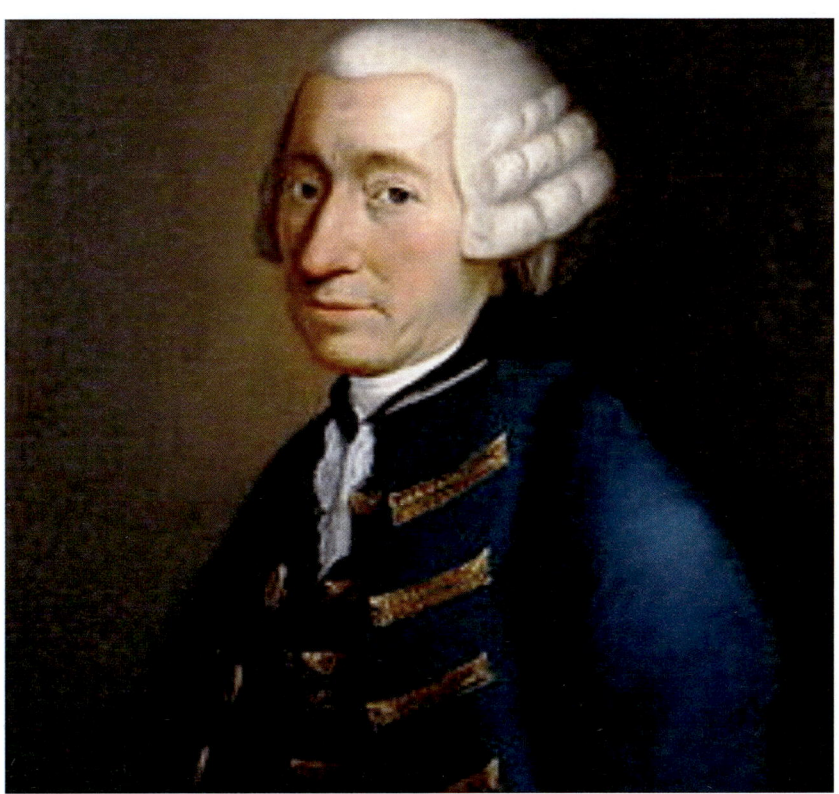

Tobias Smollett (1721 – 1771) Scottish surgeon, poet and author. Author of 'The Expedition of Humphry Clinker' (1771)

Amongst the famous visitors were Jonathan Swift, Daniel Defoe, Joseph Haydn, Alexander Pope, Dr Samuel Johnson, William Cowper and Richard Brinsley Sheridan. In 1728 John Gay gave several performances of his *'Beggar's Opera'* in the Long Room or Assembly Room on Dowry Square to a full audience [2]. Edmund Burke, who was the MP for Bristol for six years, was a visitor. Many aristocrats and bishops came to see and be seen. Visitors would sometimes hire two boats to go down the river Avon, one for themselves and the second for musicians to serenade them. Some visitors would cross the Avon by the

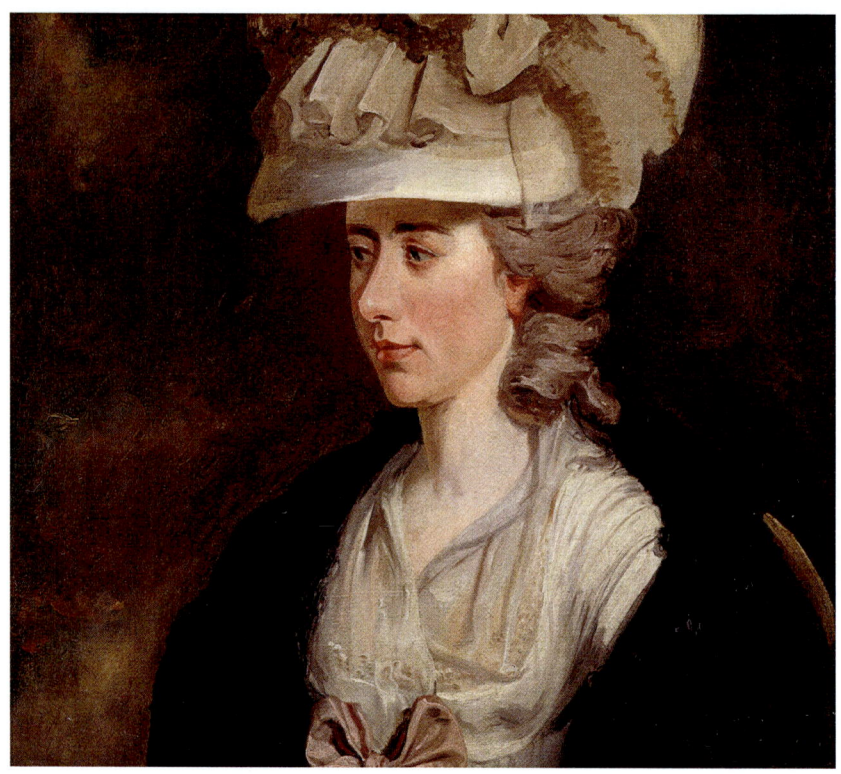

Fanny Burney (1752 – 1840) by a relative - Satirical novelist, diarist and playwright. Author of 'Evelina or the History of a Young Lady's Entrance into the World' (1778)

Rownham ferry and walk through the meadows to *'the sweet and wholesome village of Ashton'* where they would eat strawberries and cream.

Frances Sheridan, the mother of Richard Brinsley Sheridan, in her 1761 novel *'The Memoirs of Miss Sidney Bidulph'*, wrote about the *"enchanting variety of moving pictures to be seen when the ships passed close under the windows"* of the Hotwell House[6].

Tobias Smollett, a Scottish Naval Surgeon, poet and author, in his 1771 novel, *'The Expedition of Humphry Clinker'*, gives vivid descriptions of visitors to the Hotwell [7].

The satirical novelist, diarist and playwright Fanny Burney also describes the Hotwell experience in her 1778 novel *'Evelina or the History of a Young Lady's Entrance into the World'*[8]. Interestingly, later in life, aged fifty-eight, Burney gives the most riveting account of a mastectomy on record without anaesthesia[9]. This was performed in Paris in 1811 by Napoleon's surgeons Doctors Larrey and Dubois. This is one of the earliest accounts of surgery by a patient. She lived another twenty nine years, dying aged almost eighty-eight.

Diseases treated at the Hotwell

In addition to scurvy, many other conditons were thought to be helped by the Hotwell spring water. Thus *"To cure or palliate acrimonious blood, consumptions, weaknesses of the lungs, hectic fevers, uterine & other internal haemorrhages & inflammations; spitting of blood, dysentery & purulent ulcers of the viscera."*

Also diabetes mellitus, kidneys, urinary stone and gravel, old sores (applied outwardly), *"Hot livers, feeble brains & red pimply faces"*, Melancholy, skin diseases and later consumption (tuberculosis).

Various doctors insisted that all treatment should be under the professional direction of an apothecary, barber-surgeon or physician. A strict regime as shown below was the norm.

The Invalid's Day[4].

6.00am: drink asses' milk and rest for one hour in bed. If perspiration, rest on the bed lightly clad.

7.00am or earlier: Rise and go to the Hotwell.

7.30am: take first glass of water then walk for 30 minutes in the open air if weather permits or under the colonnade.

8.00am: take second glass, and then ride on horseback or in a carriage for an hour.

9.00am: breakfast followed by private avocations.

12.00 noon: take customary medicine.
1.00pm: Go to the Hotwell and drink two glasses of water.
1.30: ride on the Downs again.
4.00: Dinner and remain quiet or rest on a couch until 6.00pm.
6.30pm: Tea.
7.00pm: Walk, if unable to then ride.
9.00pm: Supper.
11.00pm Take night medicine and go bed.

So apart from drinking the Hotwell water, rest and fresh air exercise were important aspects of the treatment.

Patients and outcomes

Thomas Fuller in his Book of Worthies of England (1662) states: *"St Vincent's Well is sovereign for sores and sickness, to be washed in or drunk of.... experience proveth that beer brewed thereof is wholesome against the spleen; and Dr Samuel Ward afflicted with that malady, and living in Sidney College, was prescribed the constant drinking thereof, though it was costly to bring it through the Severn, and narrow seas to Lin (Kings Lynn) and thence by river to Cambridge"* [10].

Samuel Ward was a theologian, the Master of Sidney Sussex College and a translator of the King James Bible. He left extensive papers, which include descriptions of the aetiology and treatment of various illnesses [11]. He gives detailed lists of his symptoms at given moments. The spleen is mentioned on various occasions and he was clearly subject to digestive disorders. In 1612 he gives details of a purgative prescribed by Mr. Butler. It is likely that he got to know of the Bristol Hotwell in his capacity as Archdeacon of Taunton from 1615 onwards. He was the Master of Sidney Sussex College when Oliver Cromwell was a student there and it is likely that he taught him, as it was a small college.

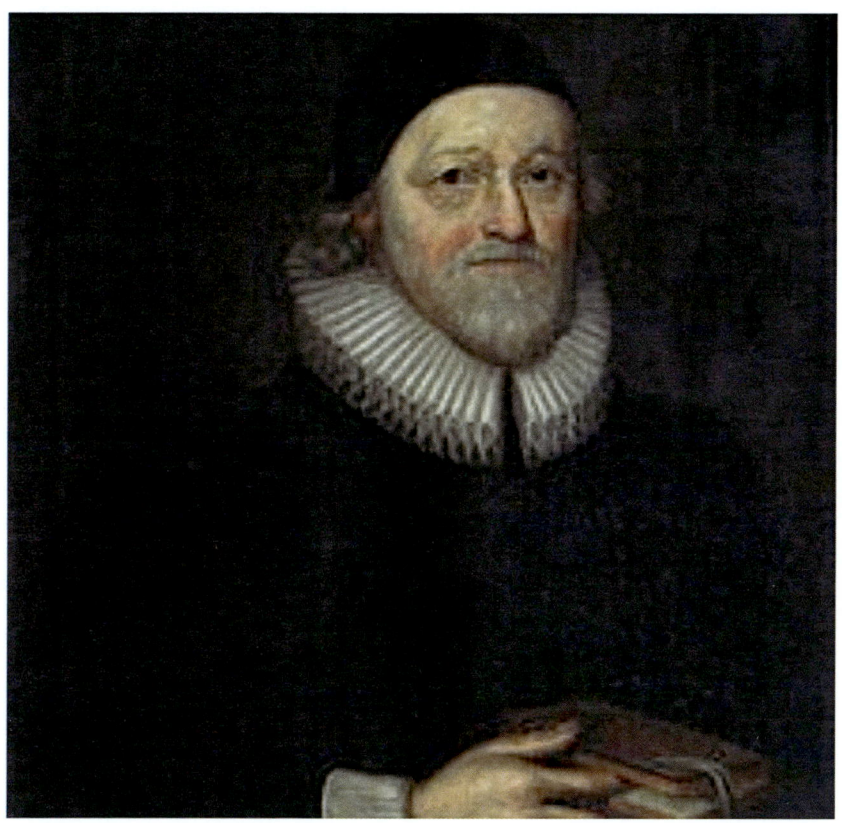

Samuel Ward (1572–1643) Theologian and Master of Sidney Sussex College. A translator of the '1611 King James Bible' and taught Oliver Cromwell

There is the 1680 famous case of *"William Gaggs a baker of Castle Green, Bristol, a very fat man, at his prime aged 38. He was seized with so violent diabetes, that he made at least 3 gallons of very sweet urine with a large quantity of oil swimming thereon every night, and could not sleep for either drinking or pissing. Which in 6 days (his appetite gone), so run off his fat and flesh that he was reduced to helpless skin and bones. Left off by his Physicians, (not sparing any money), and given over by his wife and friends for a dead man (several of his neighbours then dying of the same disease, not knowing the water's use), he resolutely cast himself on God's mercy and the Hotwell water (though ignorant of its use). Imploring his friends to support him to the Hotwell as their last case of kindness, which with difficulty they performed, he fainting every step. Yet to God's glory and their astonishment his strength so came to him with every glass, that he made them loose him. He returned home without assistance, only aided now & then with a sip of his holy water bottle. His trusty friend the Hotwell Water which instantly vanquished his insatiable thirst and stopped his pissing, and restored his depraved appetite, that at his return home, he ate a large & savoury meal, and by drinking the Water for some time, perfectly attained his former state of health in all respects, living many years after. Signed Mary Gagg, his widow"* [3]. Another account of William Gagg describes him as dreaming that he is cured by drinking the Hotwell water and so the following day goes there and is cured in a few days.

In another case from 1683 *"Mr Eaglestone, aged about 23, of Bristol College Green was afflicted with a most restless pain in his back, and difficulty of making urine. Voiding sometimes red sand, whence he concluded it was the stone (his father being tortured for many years with that disease). In a months drinking in his chamber, two quarts of Hotwell Water was cured. And nicely observing his urine as he made it in a glass, it sparkled over like the Hotwell Water, in pouring out of the bottle and as clear. It never lodging above one hour, bringing with it gravel that would presently subside in large quantity. The water sharpened his appetite, restored his sleep, fortified his retentive faculties, abated his thirst, enlivened his spirits and so effectually cured him of the gravel, that he hath been free from his paternal pains and all symptoms of the stone ever since. Signed Joseph Eaglestone"* [3.]

Another patient in 1699, *"Thomas Reynolds of Frog Lane, Bristol, mason, aged 33 had for 6 years the Kings Evil, running at a hole quite through his thigh (the scars dismal), out of which worked several bones. Amongst them one bone of an inch broad and above two inches long, smooth on the one side and like a honeycomb on the other side. After King James's* (James II, 1685-88) *fruitless touch, and the miserable cutting and slashing of the surgeons without any success. When reduced to skin and bones, and for want of food and sleep of most ghostly aspect. The constant drinking the Hotwell Water restored his lost appetite. He drank it in large quantities, and by keeping constantly wet clothes on the fistula, dipt in the same Water, he is now perfectly well and hath so been for some years past. He hath no signs, pains or breakings out of the Evil, or is troubled with any other Malady. Witness his own hand and signed Thomas Reynolds. This is a well known instance"* [3.]

According to his Journals and Letters John Wesley, aged fifty to fifty-one, attributed his sudden recovery from *"galloping consumption"* to the virtues of the Hotwell, where he could be *"Free from noise and hurry"* in 1753-4 [12,13.]

"Sat 24th Nov. 1753: I rode home, and was pretty well till night; but my cough was then worse than ever. My fever returned at the same time, together with the pain in my left breast; so that I should probably stayed at home.

Mon 26th Nov. 1753: Dr Fothergill told me plain, I must not stay in town a day longer; adding, 'if anything does thee good, it must be the country air, with rest, asses' milk, and riding daily'.

Wed 2nd Jan. 1754: I took a post-chaise, in which I reached Bristol about eight in the evening.

Fri 4th Jan: I began drinking the water at the Hot Well, having a lodging at a small distance from it.

Sun 19th March: I took my leave of the Hot Well, and removed to Bristol.

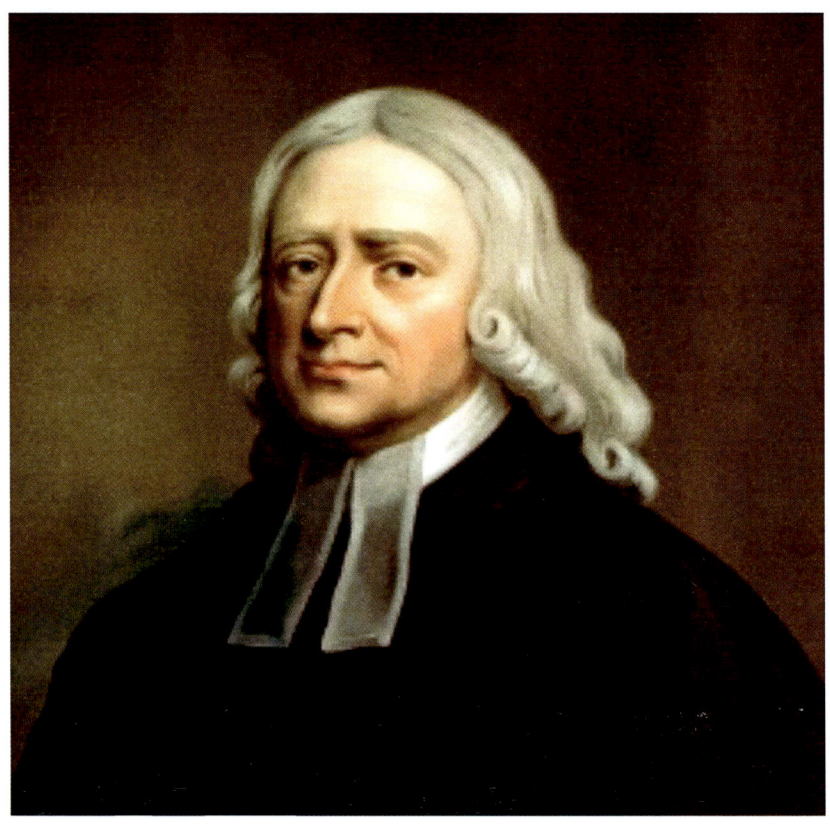

John Wesley (1703 – 1790) by George Romney. At the Hot Well 1753-1754 Author of 'Primitive Physic, or, An Easy and Natural Method of Curing Most Diseases' (1744)

Fri 9th Aug: I consulted Dr Fothergill who advised me to return to the Hot Well without delay.

Wed 14th Aug: I took lodging at the New Hot Well, where I was free both from noise and hurry, and had an opportunity of drinking the water late in the evening and early in the morning".

Dr John Fothergill FRS was a clever, eccentric Quaker physician and botanist, who in this crisis was said to have saved Wesley's life. He prescribed *'country air, with rest, asses' milk and riding daily'*, anticipating the most proved modern treatment for consumption, of which all his friends believed Wesley was actually dying. He also is known to have treated Fanny Burney. Wesley took an interest in illness and in 1744 was the author of *'Primitive Physic, or, An Easy and Natural Method of Curing Most Diseases'*

Many patients came to the Hotwell when physicians had failed. The Revd Dr Hammonds of Christ Church Oxford, sent his servant Christopher Pyman, *"After the Dr had left him past hopes of life, with his funeral directions in Bristol College Green, a dismal spectacle, wasted to the last degree in consumption at the prime of his age".*

In 1745, Dr George Randolph wrote about phthisis pulmonaria and stressed that the Hotwell water could not work miracles: *"Some come not 'til it is too late to help them; others with symptoms the water will not reach; all expecting miracles, not considering the great variety of cases comprehended under this one name, or that which might of been of service in the beginning, becomes of little or no efficacy in the later stages."* He thus showed more professional acumen and honesty than many other medical attendants.

A Hotwell guidebook wrote of physicians: *"When they find their art is ineffectual, and the case desperate, then & not till then the physician consigns his patient to the Bristol Hotwell to try the effect of the water, by which he avoids the imputation of their dying under his hands".*

In 1787 the Strangers' Burial Ground was opened as an overflow burial ground of St. Andrew's Church in Clifton. It catered for unfortunate commoners and non-parishioners, dying mainly from consumption, who were visitors to the Hotwells and came from outside the parish. The grave of Thomas Beddoes, who founded the Pneumatic Institute, is in the Strangers' Burial Ground, which was closed in 1871.

In 1807, Samuel Taylor Coleridge's Bristolian brother-in-law, the Poet Laureate Robert Southey, observed of doctors: *"They still send the paralytic to find relief at Bath, and the consumptive to die at the Hotwells."*

Decline of the Hotwell

By 1816, George III and the Prince Regent had made seaside spas like Weymouth, Brighton & Scarborough more fashionable. This and the revival of the Grand Tour after the end of the Napoleonic Wars led to the decline of the Hotwell. In 1822 the New Hotwell House was built behind the Old Hotwell House, which was then demolished. This made way for a new road which was to pass along the Hotwell end of the gorge and up the incline now known as Bridge Valley Road to Clifton. Thus the Hotwell was no longer in a cul-de-sac. At that time, there was no English city

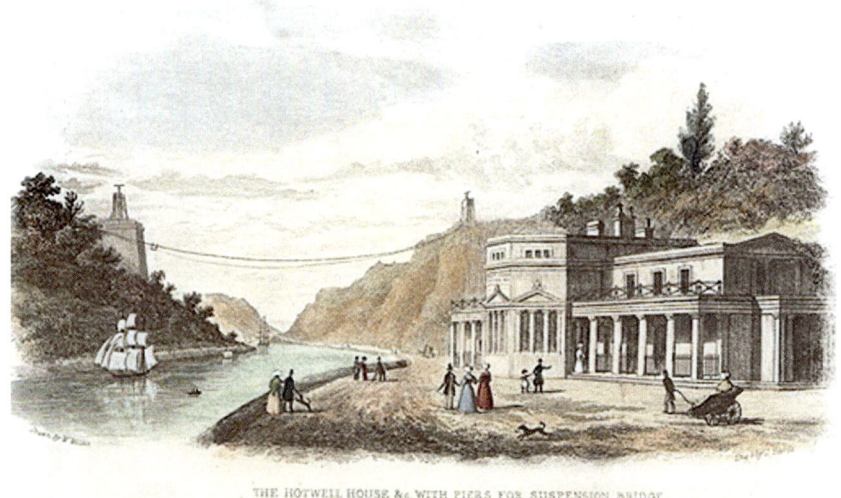

New Hotwell House (1822-1867) with piers for Suspension Bridge c1862 Designed in the Tuscan style: Royal Clifton Spa, Pump Room and Baths, Hotwells, Bristol. Royal status granted in 1851.

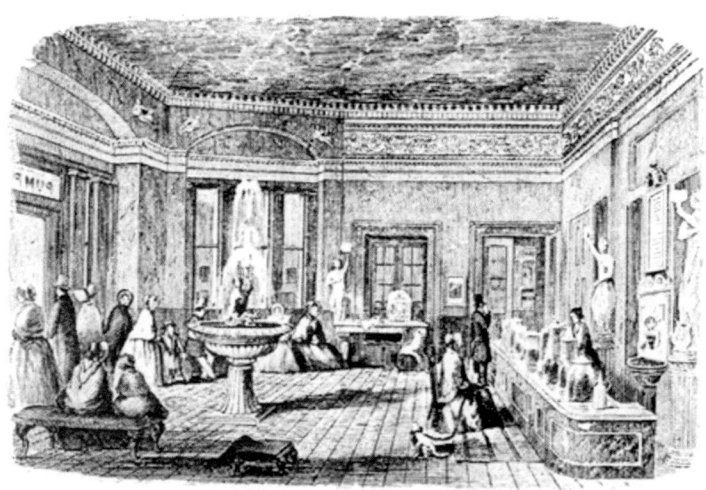

Interior of the new improved entrance hall to the Royal Clifton Spa c1851, known as the Pump Room. The Hotwell (summer) became a friendly rival to Bath (winter) as a Georgian spa.

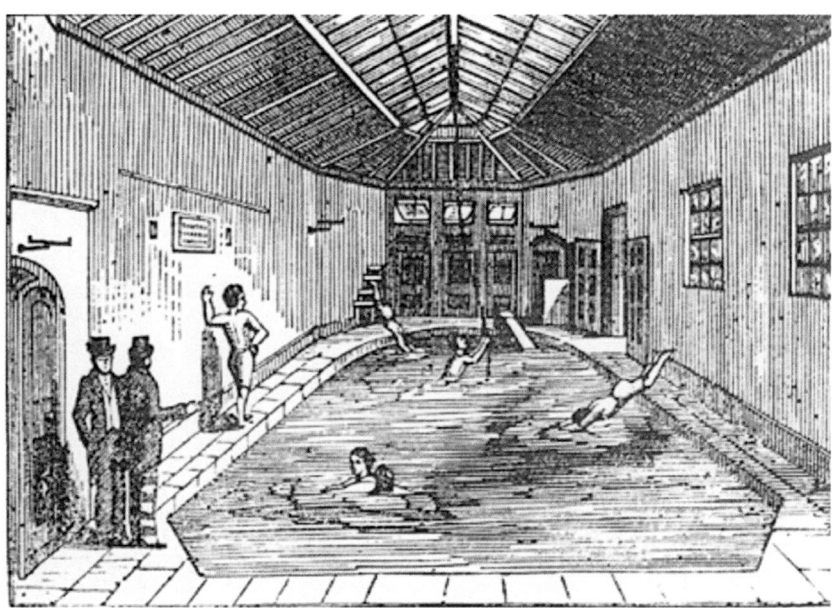

The Tepid Swimming Bath at the Royal Clifton Spa, probably first opened in 1851, demolished in 1867

outside London more attractive to artists than Bristol, and the Hotwell Spa in the Avon Gorge was seen as a major national landmark.

The New Hotwell House was built in the Tuscan style with an octagonal centre and flanking wings fronted by Tuscan porticos. It contained a Pump Room fed by the Hotwell, a fountain, statues, baths and a tepid swimming pool.
It was gas lit and provided accommodation, breakfast and dinner. By 1851 it was granted royal status and was known as Royal Clifton Spa, Pump Room, Bath and Mineral Aerated Water Manufactory.

By 1867, the Spa had declined and the New Hotwell House was demolished and the Hotwell Point removed to straighten the river, making it safer to navigate. There followed a public outcry by the people of Bristol because they had lost the Spa and the free water tap that had been one of its chief sources of early wealth and Clifton's early fashion, and which had made the city famous.

Some Observations

There is no mention of coronary heart disease at the Hotwell. Angor (angina pectoris) in the chest was depicted in accounts from ancient literature, but not described as related to coronary artery disease until the late 18th century.

There is no mention of gout at the Hotwell. This is surprising, as the first documentation of the disease is from Egypt in 2,600 BC. Historically, it was referred to as *"the king of diseases"* and *"the disease of kings"*, or *"rich man's disease"*.

Was treatment at the Hotwell effective?

Some patients and doctors thought that rest, fresh air and exercise were beneficial. Thus Wesley speaks of being *"Free *from noise & hurry"* [7]. Lydia in Smollett's Humphry Clinker describes *"This is a charming romantic place. The air is so pure, the Downs so agreeable, the furze in blossom, the ground enamelled with daisies, primroses & cowslips... the company so good-natured, so free, so easy... an enchanting variety of moving pictures."*

The status acquired by going to the Hotwell to *'take the waters'* in the invalid role may have been helpful for some patients.

We know that the Georgians drank a lot of alcohol. The Prime Minister, Pitt the Younger, was known as *'a three bottle man'* and he was said to take up to six bottles of port daily. Pitt was plagued with gout and *"biliousness"* worsened by a fondness for port, that began when he was advised to drink port to deal with his chronic ill-health. He died aged 46 in 1806, probably from stomach or duodenal peptic ulceration.

The medical historian Roy Porter says that the medical writers of Georgian England had no doubt that heavy alcohol consumption was often responsible for ill-health and disease[14]. Perhaps at the Hotwell there was decreased alcohol intake and an element of re-hydration.

In the early days of the Hotwell, when the water was being successfully pumped and bottled, it may have been unpolluted and thus a safer source of water. According to Roy Porter, many people in the eighteenth century held the *'Rational belief that all doctors would kill you, but some charged more for the privilege than others'*!

In 1912, it was found that the Hotwell water was radioactive, with a reading one hundred times higher than the normal water supply.

A revival was attempted in the latter half of the nineteenth century, with water pumped up to Clifton to the Grand Spa Hotel Pump Room with Russian and Turkish Baths. But that's another story!

References

1. Personal communication Dr Ruth Richardson FRHS, Wellcome Research Fellow in the History of Medicine at University College, London. 2016
2. Griffiths L M (1902) The Reputation of the Hotwell (Bristol) as a Health-Resort *The Bristol Medico-Chirurgical Journal Vol 20: No75.*
3. Underhill J (1703)Thermalogia Bristoliensis
4. Waite V (1960) *The Bristol Hotwell.* Bristol Branch of the Historical Association
5. Defoe D A, (1720) *A Tour through the whole island of Great Britain*
6. Frances Sheridan (1761) *The Memoirs of Miss Sidney Bidulph*
7. Tobias Smollett (1771) *The Expedition of Humphry Clinker*
8. Fanny Burney (1778) *Evelina or the History of a Young Lady's Entrance into the World*
9. http://newjacksonianblog.blogspot.com/2010/12/breast-cancer-in-1811-fanny-burneys.html
10. Fuller T (1662) *The Worthies of England*
11. Personal communication with Mr Nicholas Rogers FSA, Archivist, Sidney Sussex College, Cambridge 2018.
12. John Wesley (1753) *Journal* Vol 4
13. John Wesley (1753) *Letters* Vol 3
14. Porter R (1985) The Drinking Man's Disease: The 'Pre-History' of Alcoholism in Georgian Britain *Addiction* Vol 80, Issue 4

All I Want For Christmas Is My Two Front Teeth
LOIS M TUTTON BDS MSc
Presneted to the Society on Monday 10th Dec.2018

"All I want for Christmas is my two front teeth,
My two front teeth
See my two front teeth!
Gee, if I could only have my two front teeth,
I could wish you "Merry Christmas."
It seems so long ago since I could say
"Sister Susie sitting on a thistle!"
Gosh oh gee, how happy I'd be,
if I could only whistle......."

The novelty Christmas song above, written in 1944 by Donald Yelter Gardner (1913-2004), a teacher in Smithtown New York titles this paper. It was initially recorded by Spike Jones and his City Slickers in 1947 and reached the top of the pop charts in 1948 and 1949. It has since been recorded by numerous performers since, Gardner's favourite being the one by Nat King Cole.

Gardner was stimulated to write this from his observation that the majority of the junior class he was taking had missing front teeth! A natural phenomenon of that age group changing from the deciduous to permanent dentition. (Fig.1)

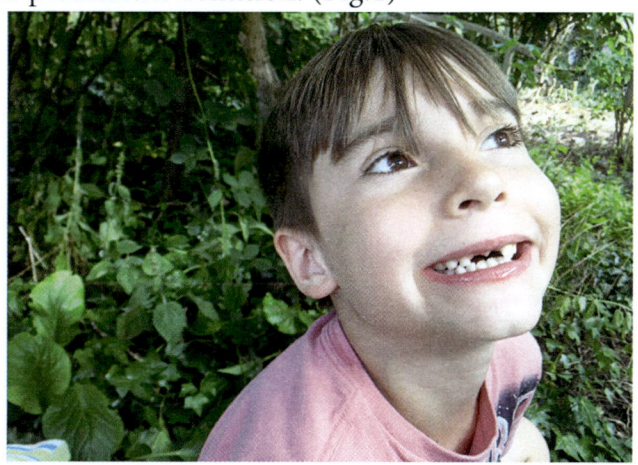

Fig 1 Typical appearance of child having lost the upper central deciduous incisors

The reality for adults who lose their front teeth from trauma or have disfigured front teeth is not so pleasant and was a permanent disfigurement. The teeth of Queen Elizabeth I were blackened stumps from caries and possibly lead poisoning and in modern times drug usage and some foodstuff dependencies lead to similar problems. (Figures 2a and b)

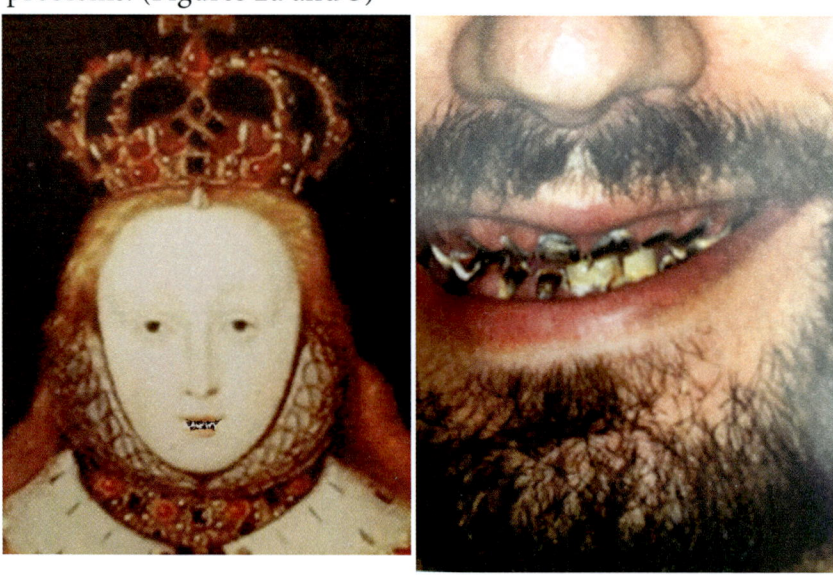

Fig.2 (a and b)
Queen Elizabeth I and her blackened stumps and a modern day example

Solutions for provision of replacement teeth have been around for centuries as shown on excavated skulls where either real teeth (Etruscans 700 BC, Egyptians 7th century and Waterloo teeth 19th century), carved wood (17th century), ivory (18th century) and porcelain (19th century) teeth have been laced together with silver or gold wire and attached to teeth adjacent to the space where teeth have been lost (Fig.3). This technique was probably not the most effective or comfortable in restoring masticatory skills, aesthetics, speech and self-esteem but the wealthy pursued such restorations as evidenced from their remains.

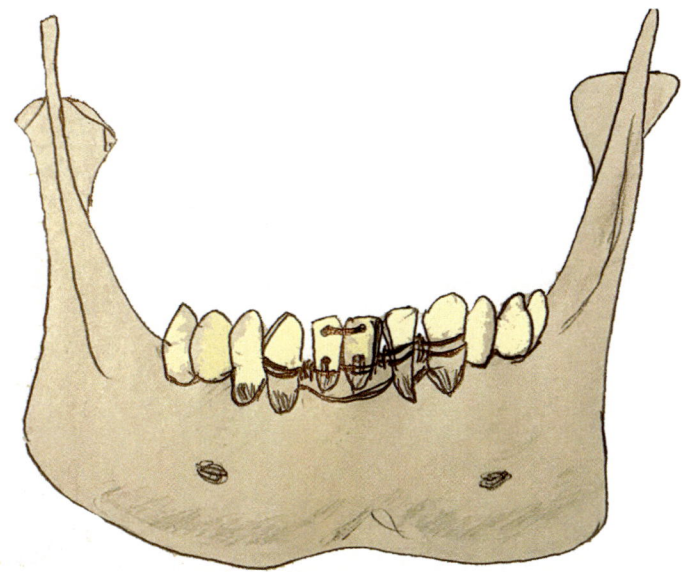

Fig.3
Bridge work found on the mandible of an Egyptian Mummy 2000 BC

The 'lost wax' or 'cire-perdue' process for casting gold and silver and other metals had been known for 6,000 years. However, the high heat involved made it difficult to combine this technique with the lower combustible materials previously described. Fixing 'teeth' in after casting and polishing a base was not easy as glues and cements and clasps were not reliable in the rigour of the oral environment. Taking impressions of the mouth was also a real problem. In the 15th century in Japan carved wooden dentures were made from beeswax impressions. In 1728 Pierre Fouchard made metal frames with teeth sculpted from animal bone. In 1770 Duchateau in France patented a technique for making dentures from porcelain. One of his apprentices, Nicholas Dubois de Chamant filed a British patent using porcelain paste from Wedgwood in 1791. In 1820 Samuel Stockton, a goldsmith perfected making porcelain dentures mounted on 18 carat gold plates. All of these dentures were of very poor fit and highly uncomfortable for the

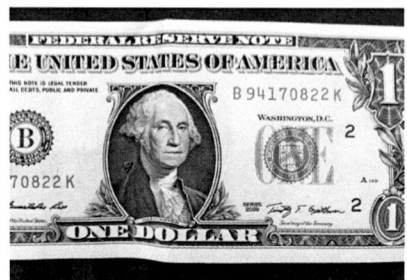 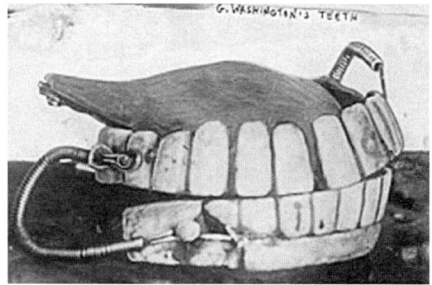

Fig 4 (a and b): George Washington and a pair of his dentures

wearer. George Washington, American President 1789-1797 was determined to restore his lost dentition and spent a small fortune having four sets made by his dentist John Greenwood. The literature is peppered with tales of his denture problems and his resultant severe portraits (Figures 4a and 4b).

Before 1851 a set of hand carved ivory dentures would cost 25 guineas and barely fit the mouth, so when Charles Goodyear experimented with adding sulphur to India rubber (caoutchouc) and heating the mixture to 115 degrees Celsius (a process called Vulcanisation) it heralded a new era for denture making. His brother Nelson founded the Goodyear Dental Vulcanite Company (GDVC) USA in 1864 and a set of dentures could be made for 6 Guineas using their patented Vulcaniser. The GDVC sold licences to dentists to use the process and the company was extremely diligent in pursuing dentists for their share of fees. In 1878 Josiah Bacon, it's Finance Officer, was shot dead by dentist Samuel Chalfant who was aggrieved at the ruthless way Bacon chased dentists for these fees. In 1881 the Goodyear patents ran out and vulcanite dentures became more readily available and cost £5. Claudius Ash used vulcanite for the bases and teeth obtained from fallen soldiers at the Battle of Waterloo (1815) and from the resurrectionists. Figures 5a, b and c show a set of vulcanite dentures with porcelain teeth which belonged to my husband's grandmother. She happily wore these for over sixty years until they could no longer be mended and she had an acrylic set made.

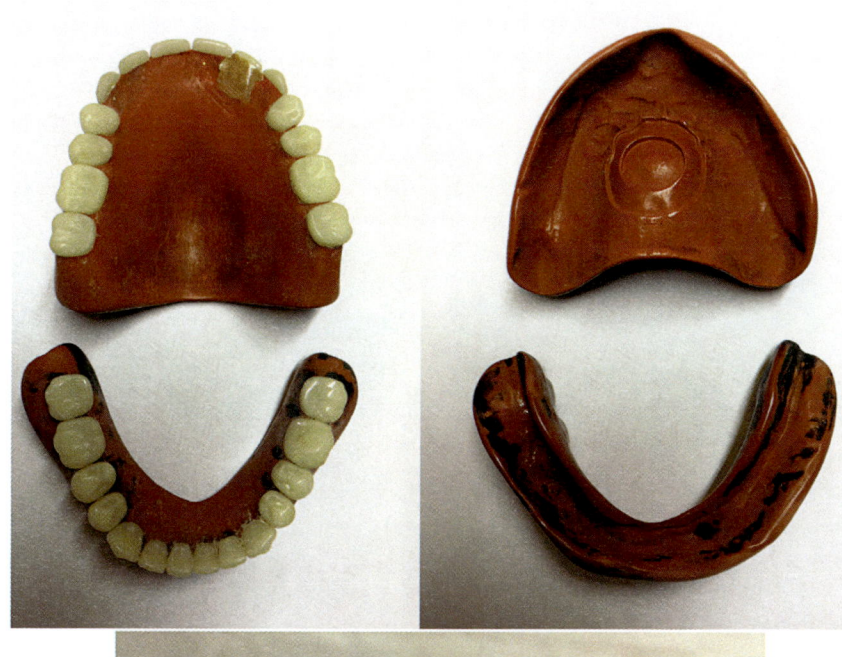
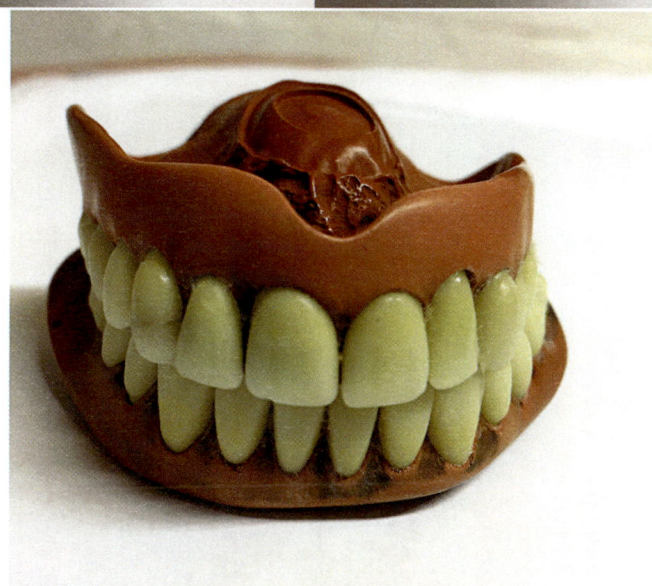

Fig 5
Gran Goddard's vulcanite dentures

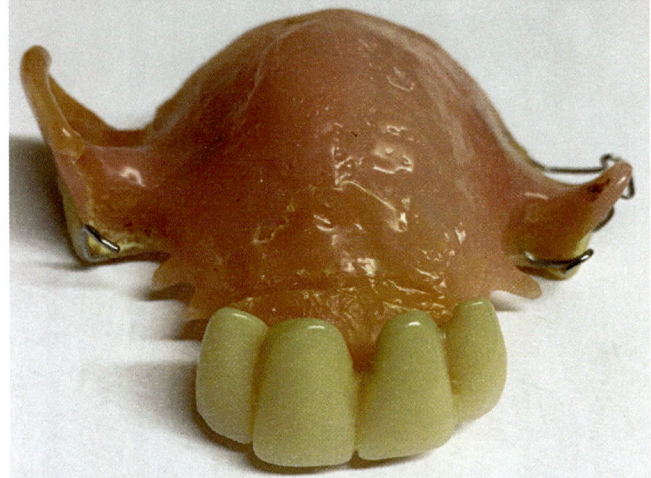

*Fig 6
An acrylic
partial denture*

Incidentally both she and the author's grandmother had all their teeth removed and dentures fitted as presents for their 21st birthdays!

Hyatt used Celluloid as a denture base in 1868 but it had an unpleasant odour from the camphor which was used as plasticiser and the material did not hold it's shape for long.

The early 20th century saw Bakelite 1909 -1939 being tried, until Acrylic (Polymethyl methacrylate) dentures superseded it in 1938 (Fig 6). Acrylic is hard, translucent and inert. It has no unpleasant odor or toxicity once processed and is relatively easy to manipulate and cheap.

The development of both general and local anaesthetics from the 1880s to present day has greatly helped to further the practice of dentistry. Most successful local anaesthetics date from 1947 onwards and have enabled painless complex procedures to be performed on teeth and when necessary, their removal.

Crowns and Bridges require the removal of tooth tissue. This process has been made easier with the development of high speed air turbine handpieces and precision made dental drill bits made of tungsten carbide, steel and diamonds. These handpieces and air rotors are driven by air compressors which need to provide clean compressed air uncontaminated with oil or water. Water is used to cool the high speed cutting of the teeth and the advent of reliable suction equipment has developed alongside that of the cutting tools.

Dental Implants made from Titanium have become possible over the last fifty years. The technique involves screwing a precision made hollow tube into the bone of the jaw, allowing it to heal and osseo-integration to take place. A preformed post is then inserted and fixed inside the tube and the superstructure acts as a former on which a crown is constructed. Such implants can be used to replace single or multiple teeth. Several implants are capable of carrying a superstructure of several teeth. This can be very successful and restores form, function and aesthetics. Interestingly Mayan skulls from 600 A.D. have been found where sea shells, carved stones (eg.jade) had been successfully embedded in the jaw to replace missing teeth and such natural materials had actually fused to the jawbone.

None of the advanced conservation/prosthetic techniques described would have been possible without improvements in impression materials. From Mid 19thC. onwards the use of flexible materials in inflexible impression trays opened the door to advance from materials such as beeswax to waxes with additives such as Plaster of Paris (gypsum), Impression compound (fatty acids, shellac, glycerine and filler), Zinc-oxide eugenol paste, hydrocolloid, agar, alginate, polysulphides, polyethers and silicones. Since the widespread development of computers, digital imaging and digital construction techniques are becoming widely available.

A smile is an important feature of the way we communicate with each other and also exercises the muscles of the face. If you have disfigured teeth due to trauma (Fig 7), caries (decay), genetic

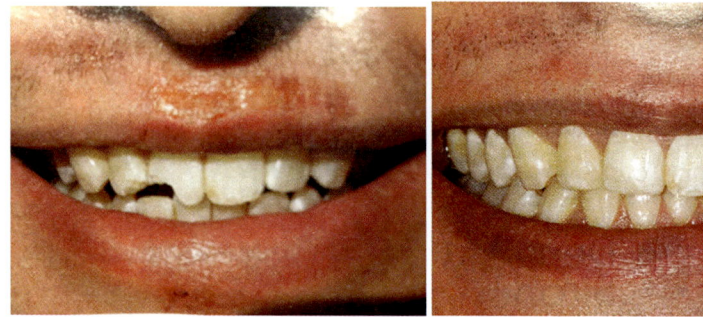

Fig 7: "I slid down the bannister as fast as I could!" (pre- and post- restoration)

and developmental abnormalities such as poor mineralisation or Fluorosis then you would try not to show your teeth and hence not smile. The great leaps forward in polymer chemistry from 1970s onwards have enabled plastics and adhesives to be developed which have toothlike properties and remain relatively inert in the unforgiving oral environment thus enabling in situ repairs and aesthetic additions to the teeth. Less tooth tissue is lost in the process than previous techniques which required considerable cutting back of tooth structure to prepare for the making of laboratory constructed crowns and bridges from precious metals and porcelain. Veneers made from porcelain or plastic can be stuck successfully to the the front surface of the teeth and in some cases a replacement tooth can be attached to an adjacent tooth or teeth without removal of any tooth tissue such as in the Rochette bridge (Fig 8).

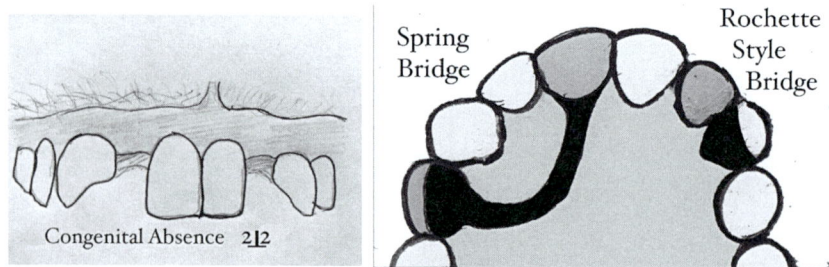

Fig 8. Example of two simple bridges to replace single missing teeth

1948 saw the start of the National Health Service (NHS) and dentistry was free for the first 4 years then a £1 flat rate patient fee was levied on each course of treatment. By 1978 the patients contribution for full dentures was £24 and, by 2018, £265.50. Private dentures can cost anything from £600 - £2000 and implants which are not available on the NHS, cost around £2000 per unit.

The author started training in dentistry in 1971 and worked in general dental practice from 1976 until 2007 and acknowledges that the explosion of improved equipment, new materials, and techniques for their use, enabled her to provide professionally satisfying dentistry restoring form, function and aesthetics to patients who would otherwise be personally and socially compromised. All these advances enable the provision of front teeth ready for a Christmas full of positive social interaction and much merrymaking!

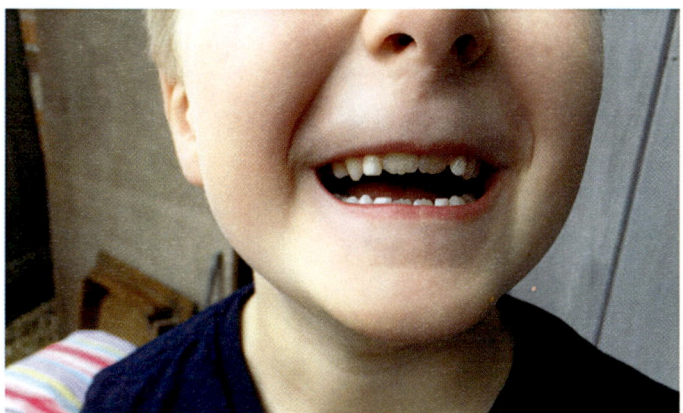

Fig 9. *The two front teeth have appeared!*

References

1. Fixed Bridge Prostheses D.H.Roberts FDS RCS Pub.John Wright and Sons Ltd.1973
2. Various Wikipedia articles
3. Celeste M Abraham A brief Perspective on Dental Implants, their surface coatings and treatments

The History of MRI
Paul R Goddard

Presented to the Bristol Medico-Historical Society 10th December 2018

A short history of magnetism

The study of magnetism has its origins back in the days of the cave men. For a very long time homonims and early humans have made stone tools. The earliest stone tools date back 3.3 million years.

An article in Nature suggests that more ancient species, such as Australopithecus afarensis or Kenyanthropus platyops may have been more sophisticated than was thought[1]. During that time the homonims must have noticed that some stones have peculiar properties of attraction and repulsion.

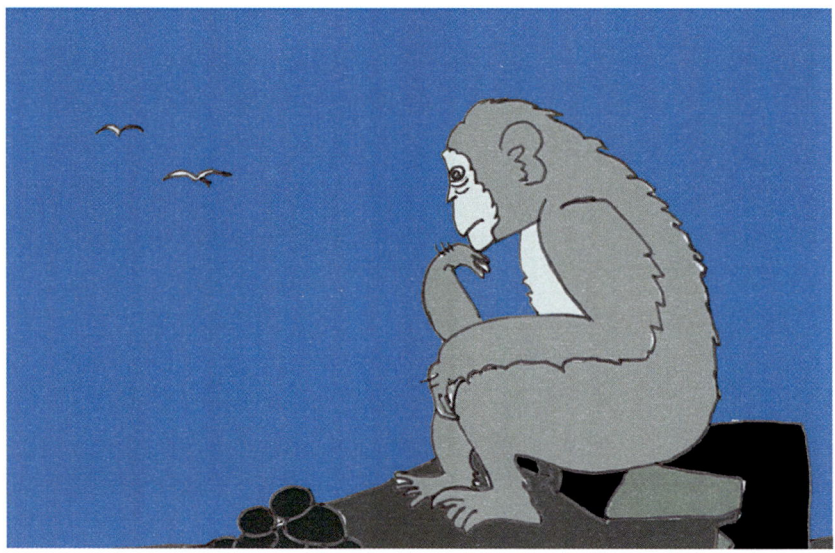

Very early hominim contemplating the usefulness of broken rocks and marvelling at some jumping stones he has discovered.

Perhaps they sat and pondered about the usefulness of such stones but maybe they were told by a tribal elder that the jumping stones were of no use and that they should get back to their work.

Lascaux Paintings

That early hominims may have discovered magnetic rocks is purely speculation. The earliest definite use of a magnetic material was as a pigment for rock paintings. The mineral Goethite (FeO(OH)[2], which is weakly magnetic, was used in the 17,300 years old cave painting of Aurochs, horses, and deer at Lascaux (photograph courtesy of Prof Saxx).[3]

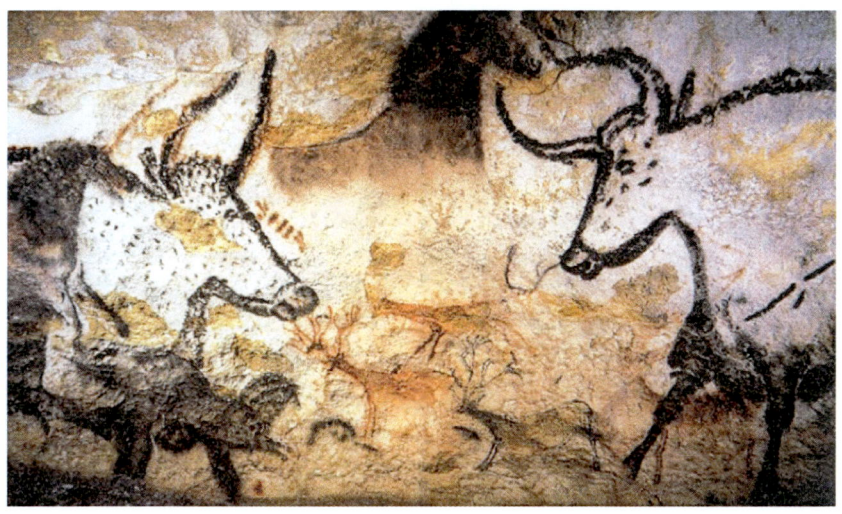

Lascaux Cave Painting (photograph courtesy of Prof Saxx)

Lodestones

Legends are recorded that *"An elderly Cretan shepherd named Magnes was herding his sheep in an area of Northern Greece called Magnesia, about 4,000 years ago. Suddenly both, the nails in his shoes and the metal tip of his staff became firmly stuck to the large, black rock on which he was standing. To find the source of attraction he dug up the Earth to find lodestones (lode means to lead or attract). Lodestones contain magnetite, a natural magnetic material Fe_3O_4. This type of rock was subsequently named magnetite, after either Magnesia or Magnes himself."*[4]

Lodestones are made of magnetite (Fe_3O_4) with inclusions of maghemite (cubic Fe_2O_3) [5].

The Chinese are reputed to have developed the mariner's compass 4,500 years ago but the first scientific report waited until the thirteenth century when Pierre Pelerin de Maricourt, a French scholar, wrote a treatise on the subject describing the polarity of magnets and the effects that magnets have on each other.[6]

Electromagnetism

In 1820 The Danish Scientist, Hans Christian Oersted, showed that passing an electric current through a wire created a deflection of a compass needle.
This was the first demonstration of electromagnetism [7].
Faraday, in England, had already created a voltaic pile. In 1821 having heard of Oersted's experiment Faraday went on to create a device that resulted in what he termed *"electromagnetic rotation"*. This was the first electric motor.[7] Oersted had shown that an electric current produced a magnetic effect. Faraday then showed that a changing magnetic current induced an electric field. This was modelled by James Clerk Maxwell as one of the four Maxwell equations which in turn became field theory.

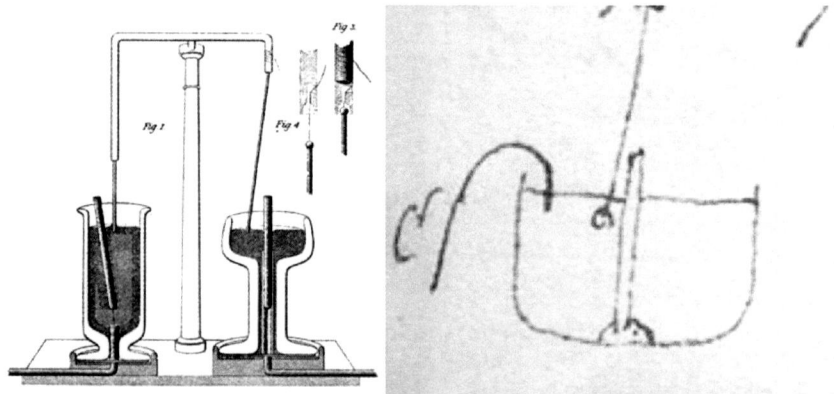

MICHAEL FARADAY's sketch of the experiment that revealed the phenomenon he called electro-magnetic rotations. The drawing is from Faraday's own notebook and is courtesy of the Royal Institution

The discovery and utilisation of magnetic resonance

In 1926 Isidor I. Rabi developed a new method of measuring the magnetic susceptibility of crystals. By 1938 he had discovered how to measure nuclear magnetic resonance and in 1944 he won the Nobel Prize.

The massive input into radar technology during WW2 provided a boost to research into Nuclear Magnetic Resonance Spectroscopy. Much of this research was carried out at the Telecommunications Research Establishment (TRE), Swanage, south-west of Poole.
This was renamed as the Royal Radar Establishment
John James, later the founder of Radio Rentals, worked on RADAR as did Jack Clemett, the father of the Bristol general practitioner Dr. Heather Sims-Williams.

Bloch and Purcell first demonstrated Nuclear Magnetic Resonance in condensed matter in 1945.The impact of NMR spectroscopy on the sciences has been substantial because of the range of information and the diversity of samples, including solutions and solids.

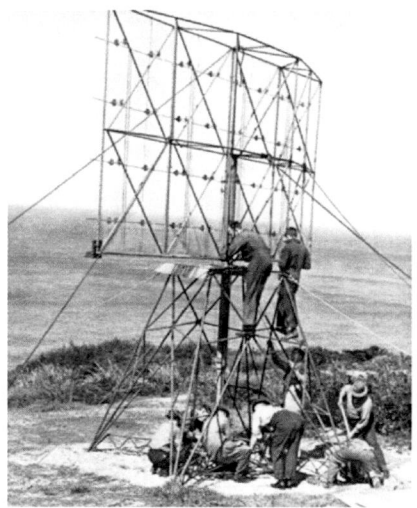
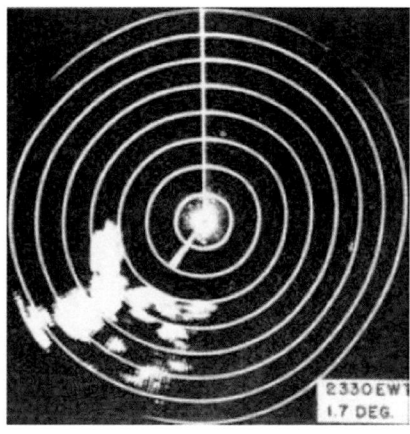

World War Two Radar

The Development of MRI

The development of MRI was spearheaded by three interesting characters.

Firstly there was Raymond Damadian. Born in Manhattan in 1936, he qualified as a doctor (MD) in 1960 and decided to go into research. He was undoubtedly the first to suggest that NMR spectroscopy could be used in the living patient and to demonstrate changes in the relaxation times, T1 and T2, in cancerous tissue compared with normal tissue.

Controversially, however, the Nobel Prize for medicine and physiology, 2003, went to Paul Lauterbur of the USA, a chemist who had initially ridiculed Damadian's ideas, and to Peter Mansfield of the UK, a physicist who did much of the work to enable slice selection in MRI and also developed echo-planar imaging.

Other British researchers who did a lot to establish MRI include John Mallard, Graeme Bydder, Iain Young, Brian Worthington and Donald Longmore.

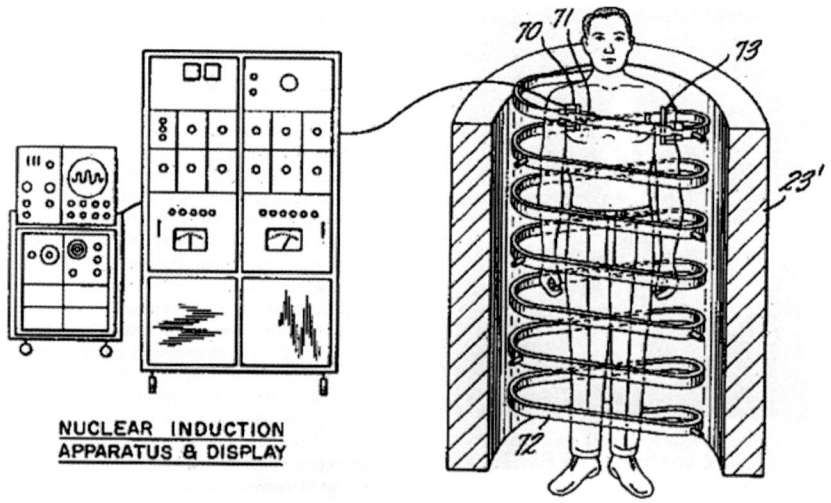

A sketch of Damadian's early equipment for in vitro NMR

A simple introduction to MRI physics.

The physics of MRI is complicated but it can be easily understood if it is considered in the following way:

- The patient lies in a large magnet
- Radio waves are passed in
- They resonate with free protons
- Radio waves pass out from the patient
- The signal is detected by receiver coils
- A picture is created on the basis of frequency and phase

Changing the timing of input and collection can alter the images, highlighting various magnetic properties such as T1 time, T2 time, Proton Density, Susceptibility etcetera. These will not be discussed in depth in this article.

The various uses of MRI

MRI can be used in all parts of the head, body and limbs. The major use of the time on the machines in the UK is within the Central Nervous System (the brain and spine) and with orthopaedic problems. MRI and MRS can be excellent at staging and studying oncology and there is a growing use in this area. MRI has been used successfully to study the heart, lungs, abdomen and pelvis.

Unfortunately the availability of MRI in the UK is ranked 31st out of 36 comparable nations and there is a similar lack of computed tomography (CT) facilities (35th out of 37). This is one of the reasons that our cancer survival rate is poor.[8]

Conclusion

This article discusses the advent of MRI. For further information on MRI in Bristol there are many articles in previous issues of the *Bristol Medico Chirurgical Journal* and its successor the *West of England Medical Journal*. In 1988 an entire issue of the *Bristol Medico-Chirurgical Journal* was dedicated to the subject.

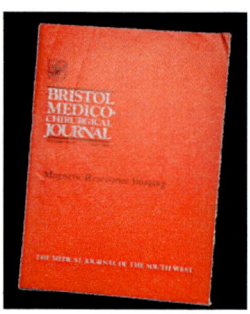

Magnetic Resonance Imaging is an astonishingly successful technique which was partially developed in the UK. It is very sad to see that the availability of MRI and CT via the British NHS lag so far behind many other nations.

References

1. 3.3-million-year-old stone tools from Lomekwi 3, West Turkana, Kenya Sonia Harmand et al 310-315 NATURE VOL 521 21 MAY 2015
2. https://en.wikipedia.org/wiki/Goethite
3. https://en.wikipedia.org/wiki/Lascaux
4. http://www.howmagnetswork.com/history.html
5. https://en.wikipedia.org/wiki/Lodestone.
6. https://en.wikipedia.org/wiki/Petrus_Peregrinus_de_Maricourt
7. https://en.wikipedia.org/wiki/Michael_Faraday#/media/File:Faraday_magnetic_rotation.jpg
8. Daily Telegraph 27th Nov 2018

The Poppy, Panacea and Plague

GORDON M STIRRAT MA, MD, FRCOG
Emeritus Professor of Obstetrics & Gynaecology, University of Bristol
Presented to the Bristol Medico-Historical Society 11 March, 2019

A Reflective Journey – Part 1

As an obstetrician I am familiar with the use of opiates in the form of, for example, pethidine, morphine or diamorphine (heroin) that have been commonly used to provide pain relief in labour for many years. It is not the purpose of this paper to discuss their effectiveness (open to question) or side effects for mother and baby (potentially serious) when used therapeutically but, rather to look briefly at the historical abuse of opiates in society and, in part 2, review what has come to be known as the 'opioid epidemic' in the 21st century. This reflective journey has been greatly enhanced by two excellent but different books – Lucy Inglis's *'Milk of Paradise – a History of Opium'*[1] and Chris McGreal's *'American Overdose – the Opioid Tragedy in Three Acts'*[2] to which I will be making fairly frequent reference in parts 1 and 2 respectively. My account is not intended to be definitive or comprehensive but rather to highlight issues on which I wish you to reflect as I have done.

Introduction

An opiate is a drug derived from opium of which the major members are morphine, codeine and thebaine. Chemically they are 'alkaloids'. They are often (particularly in the United States) misnamed 'narcotics' which includes cocaine. Table 1 lists some of the effects of opiates that illustrate their attractions and hazards. They are, of course, highly

Table 1: Effects of Opiates

Among these are:	
Pain perception decreased ++	Euphoria
Altered consciousness	Reduction of fear
Some respiratory depression	and apprehension,
Cough reflex decreased	Lessening of inhibitions
Vomiting +	'Feeling good'

addictive and this is a major problem that has been associated with their use throughout history that will be discussed later.

The term 'Opioid' refers to all natural and synthetic alkaloids that bind to specific receptors in the brain. The physiological purpose of these receptors is to bind naturally occurring endorphins, small chains of amino acids produced by the pituitary gland and hypothalamus to produce pain relief and a sense of well-being. The name derives from 'endogenous morphine' i.e. internally produced morphine.

Opioids are generally used for relief of moderate and severe pain that does not respond to standard painkillers. The advice is that they should be prescribed for a limited time mainly due to the risk of addiction (though this should not prevent primary prescription when clinically indicated). The predominant legal uses for opioids today are for relief of acute pain (particularly following surgery), during labour and, as we shall see, in terminal care. Their role in the management of chronic pain is very controversial and this is a major theme of these reflections. In addition to the opiates mentioned above the opioids most commonly used currently include methadone, tramadol, fentanyl and alfentanil.

Whereas endorphins are quickly cleared from their brain receptors, opioids bind to then more avidly with the result that their effects are more potent and long-lasting, some more so than others [e.g. fentanyl is 100 times more potent than morphine].

The Poppy as Panacea and Plague:

The story starts with the Opium Poppy, Papaver somniferum, originally found in Turkey and named by Carl Linnaeus 250 years ago.

The narcotic and sleep-producing qualities of the poppy have been known to humankind throughout recorded history. Sumerian records from ancient Mesopotamia [5000 to 4000 BC] refer to the poppy, and medicinal reference to opium is contained in Assyrian medical tablets. Among the many things attributed to the Swiss physician, alchemist, and astrologer known as Paracelsus [1493-1541] is the reintroduction of opium to Western Europe and the introduction of laudanum, a tincture of opium heated with alcohol[3] which he made into pills that he referred to as his *'stone of immortality.'*

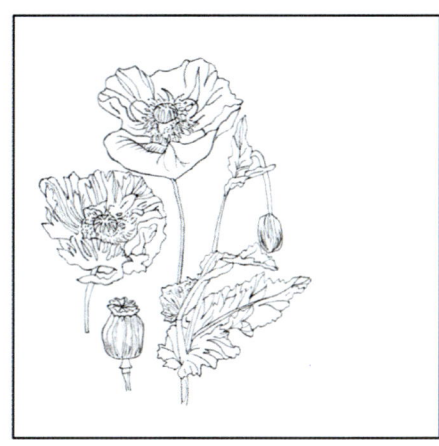

Figure 1
The Opium Poppy by Ella Cudmore

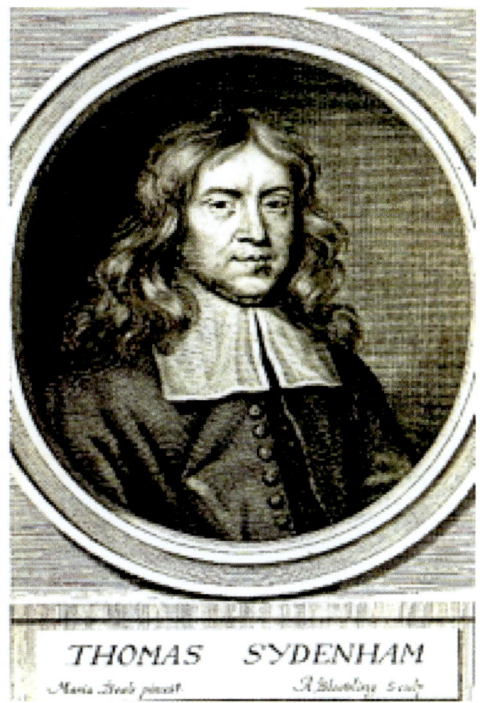

Figure 2: Thomas Sydenham

As Inglis points out *'Laudanum marked a moment of huge change for opium consumption'* [4] aided by the publicity it achieved through the concurrent development of printing. The demand for opium was firmly entrenched in Europe by the middle of the 16th century and throughout British society by the end of the 18th century, one of the significant contributors to that being Thomas Sydenham [1624-89]. He strongly promoted the use of opium for many ordinary ailments and considered that *'of all the remedies it has pleased Almighty God to give man to relieve his suffering, none is so efficacious as opium'* [4].

In 1804 Friedrich Sertürner a German pharmacist, identified the psychoactive substance secreted by the opium poppy and called it *'Morphium'* better known to us as Morphine. This was not only the first alkaloid to be extracted from opium, but the first ever alkaloid to be isolated from any plant[5].

According to Inglis [4] *'Morphine heralded a new era in drug manufacture and consumption --- It produced miraculous results instantly and* **appeared to have no side effects'** (my bold italics); but *'by the 1840s Western doctors realised that there was a dreadful problem with this wondrous new cure'* namely addiction.

The American Civil War [1861-1865][4] involved massive fatalities and appalling injuries on both sides. In 1865 the Union Army alone issued an incredible ten million opium pills and 2.8 million ounces of other opiates (mainly morphine). Thus one legacy of the excessive use of opiates during the Civil War was up to 300,000 opiate addicts[4] and morphine addiction became known as *'the army disease'*. A significant factor in the administration of such large quantities of morphine was the use of the hypodermic syringe invented, as we know it, in 1844[4] and used widely in Europe and the USA. Although this had advantages by 1880 it was realised that *'no therapeutic discovery ... has been so great a blessing and so great a curse to mankind as the hypodermic injection of morphia'* [6].

Although opium usage had begun to decline in the USA by 1914[7], in 1911 Dr. Hamilton Wright, their first Opium Commissioner (without producing evidence for his claim) that *'of all the nations of the world, the United States consumes most habit-forming drugs per capita. Opium, the most pernicious drug known to humanity, is surrounded, in this country, with far fewer safeguards than any other nation in Europe'*. This led to the so called Harrison Narcotics Tax Act (1914) to regulate and tax the production, importation, and distribution of opiates and coca products[7]. The courts interpreted this to mean that physicians could prescribe narcotics to patients in the course of normal treatment, but not for the treatment of addiction and, indeed, the importation of heroin for any purpose was banned in 1924. It is suggested that the act also marks the beginning of the creation of the modern, criminal drug addict and the American black market for drugs.

Inglis[4] describes graphically how, why and with what serious effect the use/abuse of opiates became endemic in Britain affecting all strata of society.

'The Picture of Dorian Gray' (Oscar Wilde 1891) describes opium

dens *'where one could buy oblivion, dens of horror where the memory of old sins could be destroyed by the madness of sins that were new.'* [10] Rushton[10] tells us *'Before the 1868 Pharmacy Act barbers, confectioners, ironmongers, stationers, tobacconists, wine merchants all sold opium. It was easy to come by and many people took it, including numerous authors, such as Elizabeth Barrett-Browning, Lord Byron, Wilkie Collins, George Crabbe, Charles Dickens, John Keats, Percy Bysshe Shelley, and Walter Scott'.* Samuel Taylor Coleridge and Thomas de Quincey both began misusing laudanum as teenagers. Both were friends and patients of Bristol's Thomas Beddoes [1760-1808] (he of the Pneumatic Institute). Coleridge composed his famous poem *'Kubla Khan'* in 1797 following an opium inspired dream and de Quincey being famous for his *'Confessions of an English Opium-Eater'* (1821)[4]. Both died as addicts.

The use of opium in various forms as a panacea became very common and persistent. It was routinely prescribed to both children and adults for many ailments including sleeplessness, a troublesome cough, the hiccups, headache, wind, diarrhoea, toothache, teething and dropsy to name but a few![11] Thomas Dover [1660 -1742], who trained as a physician under Thomas Sydenham and started practice in Bristol in 1682, published the recipe for his opium based *'Dover's Powder'* in 1729 that was used in the UK as a general panacea until after WW2 (and not banned in India until 1994)[4]. Paregoric (camphorated tincture of opium) was a popular over the counter treatment for diarrhoea, coughs and pain relief until well into the 20th century[4]. The so-called *'Mrs. Winslow's Soothing Syrup'* was developed in the USA in 1845 and widely marketed there and in the UK particularly *'to quiet restless infants and small children especially for teething'*. It contained a potentially lethal amount of morphine sulphate and, although in 1911 the American Medical Association linked its use to a large number of infant deaths, it was not withdrawn from sale until 1930.[8]

This was neither the first nor last time that pecuniary interests would drive the marketing and spread of the use of opiates. A major and utterly shameful example was the manner in which the British East India Company (BEIC) used the manufacture and sale of opium in India and China to make massive fortunes for many individuals who became very powerful. These included Robert Clive, 1st Baron Clive of Plassey who became obscenely rich. A chronic user of laudanum, he died in 1774 at his home in Berkeley Square, London following an overdose. It is almost unbelievable that Britain, through its surrogate the BEIC, fought two wars [1839 to 1842 and 1856 to 1860] with China in order to maintain and prosper this lethal trade. Inglis[4] tells the full story of the role of the BEIC in the opium trade and the First and Second Opium Wars. By 1906 an estimated twenty-five per cent of Chinese men at all levels of society were users and addicts[4]. In a debate in the House of Commons in 1889, Samuel Smith, the liberal MP for Flintshire declaimed:

'The gigantic evil of this opium trade is England's greatest national sin.

I am quite aware that within the last few years a feeble and a futile effort has been made to persuade the British public that the use of opium is not noxious, that opium is a comparatively healthy drug, and that it may be used by the great mass of the Chinese without any greater harm than results from the use of beer by our population, or even with any greater harm than from tobacco smoking. I have never come across a single disinterested witness who did not regard the common use of opium as one of the most terrible curses that could befall humanity.' [9]

Attempts to control the lucrative trade in opium were protracted and convoluted with vested interests persistently trying to thwart regulation. For example, Britain's involvement in the Indian opium trade with China through the 19th century was not brought to an end until the Anglo-Chinese Opium Agreements (1907-14)[11]. Suffice it to say here that the use of opiates had declined after the 1868 and 1908 Pharmacy Acts the first of which restricted opium sales to pharmacies while the second moved opiates (and cocaine) into part one of the poisons schedule[11]. The International Opium Convention at The Hague in 1912, to which Britain was a signatory, was the first global attempt at drug control and aimed to reduce the use of morphine and cocaine by restricting the manufacture of, trade in, distribution and use of, these drugs to *'legitimate'* scientific and medical purposes only. Concerns about drug misuse (particularly cocaine and opioids) among soldiers in the WW1 led to the prohibition in 1916 of the gift or sale of cocaine and opiates except on prescription. This was the first time that a doctor's prescription was required by law for the purchase of specified drugs. The first Dangerous Drugs Act that laid the foundation of further legislation and control policy in Britain was passed in 1920[12].

The 2012 BMA publication of *'Drugs of dependence: the role of medical professionals'* [12] describes the growth of drug use in Britain and the heroin crisis of the 1960s. This resulted in the Dangerous Drugs Act [1967] the two main effects of which were the restriction of the prescribing of heroin for management of addiction to doctors licensed by the Home Office and the setting up of drug treatment centres being headed by consultant psychiatrists. Methadone had recently been developed in the USA and its oral use soon replaced heroin to manage opioid addiction in the UK.[12] This is the context in which I began my training in Obstetrics and Gynaecology as is discussed below.

Part 2: Personal Reflections

London (1970-75) and Bristol (1982 -)

Having graduated from, and begun my training in, Glasgow we moved to London in 1969. I was appointed as a lecturer/senior registrar in obstetrics and gynaecology at St Mary's Hospital in 1970. There I had my first experience of the management of drug dependency in pregnancy and was struck by the commitment of the social workers and midwives involved in caring from them. Personally I had to adjust my management strategies to cope with them not telling me the truth about anything. Thus I learned the necessity of not being judgemental. The drugs they misused cross the placenta freely and affect the fetus directly. In addition to being less likely to seek antenatal care, drug dependency and its associated health and social problems can have serious effects on the unborn child such as intrauterine growth restriction and pre-term birth. The most harrowing thing is the devastating effects on the new born baby of sudden withdrawal of the drugs at birth (the oddly named *'Neonatal Abstinence Syndrome'* or NAS) leading to, among other things, irritability, high-pitched crying, increased muscle tone, seizures, poor feeding, vomiting and diarrhoea[13.]

Unfortunately there was a new epidemic of heroin abuse in the 1980s. It was accepted that these *'problem drug users'* also suffered from social, economic and other medical problems. Management was no longer seen as the sole province of the specialist clinic and, with strict safeguards, there was an increasing role for doctors outside the specialist treatment services[12].

I moved on to Oxford in 1975 and then to Bristol in 1982 to take up the chair in Obstetrics & Gynaecology. Around 1985, I established the first antenatal clinic in the South West for women dependent on drugs. Once more the commitment of the Bristol Drugs Project team, social workers and midwives was (and still is) exemplary. Case studies 1 and 2 briefly describe anonymously two case histories that greatly affected me at the time:

- Case Study 1: AH and BH, a couple in their mid to late twenties. They had become drug dependent while at university and firmly believed that it was we non-drug users who were out of line. AH was now pregnant but refused any treatment. She went into pre-term labour and delivered a 'small for dates' baby girl who then suffered from the most severe NAS I had seen. She was in the Special Care Baby Unit for many weeks. I have no knowledge as to what happened to mother, father or baby thereafter but cannot be optimistic about the outcome.

- Case Study 2: MD was a woman in her 30s with a longstanding opioid drug habit. She had sought treatment from the Bristol Drug Project Team and seemed to be doing well. She became pregnant and attended our clinic regularly. She delivered a baby boy at term and there were few problems. We felt fairly confident that she was no longer using drugs. She left Bristol and went back to her parents' home in Somerset. About a year later we learned that she had died from a heroin overdose.

It is hopefully encouraging that the numbers of women seen within the clinic have been steadily declining with 68 in 2009 and 40 in 2018. The drug usage picture is complex but use of heroin has fallen and that of cocaine increased. Some women are now being seen who, having been prescribed long-term opioids, wish to discuss the pregnancy effects and risk of NAS[14].

Personal Reflection – Oxford 1975-1982

As noted above, in 1975 I moved from London to Oxford as Clinical Reader and Honorary Consultant in Obstetrics & Gynaecology. There are two doctors from that period in my life who are part of the story I wish to tell. In 1976 Dr Robert Twycross was appointed Medical Director of Sir Michael Sobell House, the Oxford hospice, and we became friends. His contribution to the field of palliative care has been immense[15]. Dr Jane Ballantyne was training as an anaesthetist during my time in Oxford and she was known to me in that context. In 1990 she moved to Harvard University to work in Pain Medicine.

In 1971 Dame Cicely Saunders had appointed Robert Twycross to research the most effective use of opiates in relieving pain while preserving the terminally ill patient's quality of life. The work he did to standardize and simplify the treatment of their chronic pain was a major step forward in their care[15]. According to McGreal[16] in the early 1970s a small Scottish pharmaceutical company developed a slow release formula for several drugs. Saunders and Twycross asked them to make a slow-release morphine pill which they did. Called *'MST'*, it provided 8-12 hours of pain relief which was, and remains, a great step forward in the care of terminally ill patients. The Scottish company was a subsidiary of a much larger enterprise in England and the USA in particular. A few years later MST was licensed in the United States as MS Contin and, in 1984, two American doctors, Kathleen Foley and Russell Portenoy, introduced the work of Saunders and Twycross to the United States. They took things further than just for the care of the terminally ill and advocated their use they for the millions of people living with chronic pain arguing that people had a human right to be pain free.

In 1986 they reviewed thirty-eight cancer patients who had used opioids for several years[16]. They found that thirty-seven per cent still had troublesome pain and daily life was not improved but they claimed it was safe because only two patients became addicted and *'probably because they had previously abused drugs'*. The review was submitted to the journal Pain who rejected it as being flawed.

Despite protests they changed their mind on appeal and, according to McGreal[16] *'This paper marked the start of a revolution that turned attitudes to opioids on their head and brought about a fundamental shift in medical culture.'* McGreal[17] has charted a timeline of the components and disastrous effects of this revolution and table 2 outlines some of these.

Table 2: Timeline of US opioid crisis[17]

1996	The new powerful opioid pill, Oxy-Contin is released and marketed as the new hope for millions of Americans with chronic pain. It is claimed (with no evidence!) that the drug is less addictive and more effective than other narcotic painkillers. The American Pain Society, introduces the concept of *"Pain as the 5th Vital Sign"*.
1999	A sharp rise in opioid drug overdoses is recorded in West Virginia
2001	A warning is sounded that OxyContin is devastating communities in parts of Virginia, Kentucky, and West Virginia. US hospitals are required 'to prioritize pain treatment' in order to be accredited
2003	The New England Journal of Medicine publishes an article by Dr. Jane Ballantyne who was trained in Oxford and now at Harvard Medical School who was by then one of the United States' leading pain specialists. She warns that opioid painkillers do not work as long-term treatment and may even make a patient's condition worse. She is not the first or the last authoritative physician to do this but, despite strong supportive evidence, not only were all their warnings dismissed as extreme but serious attempts were made to have her sacked and struck off the medical register.
2005	Pharmaceutical companies set up *'the Pain care Forum'* to shift the focus from addiction to a claimed 'epidemic of untreated pain'.
2009	Drug overdose deaths exceed those by traffic accidents for the first time in the USA
2011	The Centers for Disease Control warns that there is an epidemic of opioids addiction
2013	Coroners started to record the first deaths from Fentanyl (100 times more powerful than morphine.)
2016	Fentanyl causes more than 20,000 deaths overtaking those from heroin and prescription opioids

Derived from official statistics Figure 3 shows the shocking picture of the situation in the USA in 2016/17 . The USA consumes more than eighty per cent of the world's opioids painkillers yet accounts for less than five percent of its population. Tragically prescription painkillers have already claimed more than a quarter of a million American lives: opioids now kill more people in the United States each year than AIDS at its most destructive and all the American soldiers who died in the Vietnam War[16]. This is compounded by a second wave of heroin and synthetic opioids such as fentanyl. A former head of the FDA has described it as *'one of the greatest mistakes of modern medicine.'* [16,19]

Figure 3

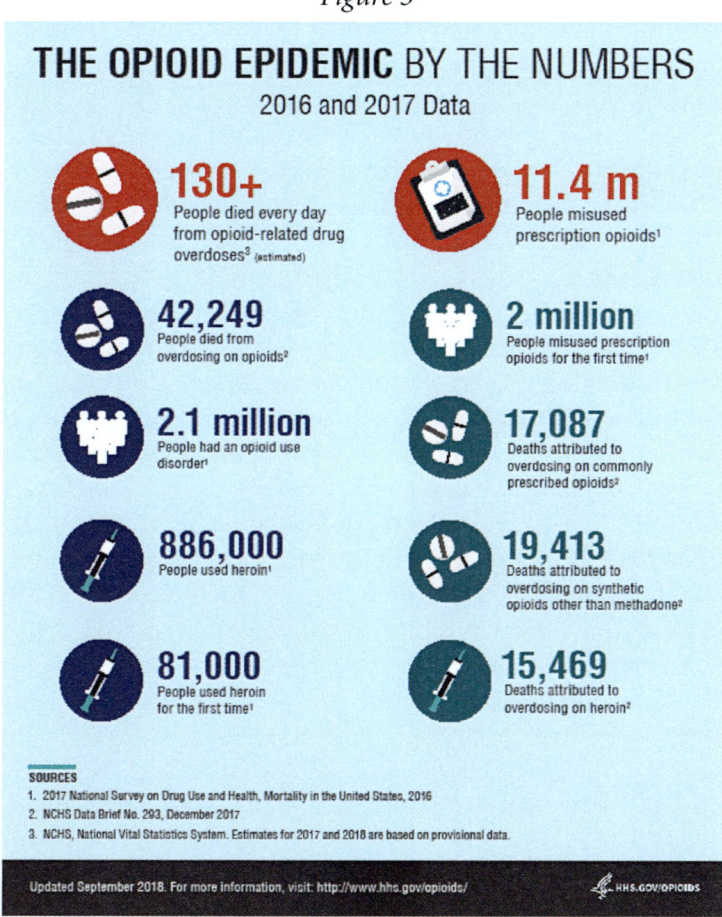

As a result of his comprehensive analysis McGreal[16] considers that this tragedy is due to *'the capture of medical policy by corporations and the failure of American institutions to protect the public'* that came about because of *'a medical system run not as a service for the public good but as a business for corporate profit'*.

We in the UK must not be complacent. Nearly twenty-four million prescriptions for opioids (particularly tramadol) were issued in 2017, ten million more than in 2007. Deaths involving opioids have more than doubled since 2012 in England and Wales, driven by a surge in heroin use [20]. Scotland has the highest reported drug-related death rate in the European Union with more than half of overdoses involving morphine or heroin[16]. As recently as 28th September 2019 the Times revealed that online pharmacies are prescribing powerful opioids without consulting GPs in breach of new regulations[21]. The UK government has ordered Public Health England to conduct a review of the scale and nature of the problem with prescription levels.

We must not let this man-made tragedy undermine the very great therapeutic benefit of opioids when used appropriately (e.g. post-operatively and for acute pain). In relation to long-term pain, according to the UK Faculty of Pain Medicine[22] there is evidence that *'opioids may reduce pain for some patients in the short and medium term (usually less than 12 weeks) for a number of chronic painful conditions'* though they accept that the research is fraught with difficulties. They suggest that *'there should be no trial of traditional opioids in chronic pain beyond modest doses over about 2-4 weeks and the therapeutic trial should be informed by important practice points'* such as - patients who do not achieve useful pain relief within 2-4 weeks are unlikely to gain benefit in the long term: short-term efficacy does not guarantee it long-term: there is no evidence for efficacy of high dose opioids in long-term pain.[22]

In conclusion, there is yet another side to the story. Commenting on a 2018 report by the Lancet Commission on Global Access to Palliative Care and Pain Relief[23] Diederik Lohman[24], from Human Rights Watch, is quoted as saying that *'the tough international rhetoric on opioids has led in some countries to opiophobia... an irrational fear around the use of these medications'*. In the Lancet Commission's analysis of opioid pain relief in different countries they conclude that whereas the USA gets thirty times more opioid pain relief medication than it needs, Mexico, China, India and Nigeria, get only 36, 16, 4 and 0.2 per cent respectively of what they need. The report calls for new methods to measure health progress that include suffering, and for the inclusion of palliative care as part of the universal health insurance governments offer their citizens. It also calls for the establishment of a clear accountability process to measure progress toward closing the pain relief gap[23].

Here I have been able to tell only part of the story of both the abuse and underuse of opioids. I have learned several important lessons during my career and from my reading – among them are the power that opiates/opioids hold over our brains and the physical and social mayhem caused by addiction; the manner in which their benefits can be turned into disaster when commercial interests are allowed free rein and the inability of some regulatory authorities to protect the vulnerable. I will leave you to draw such further conclusions as you wish.

References:

1. Inglis I: "Milk of Paradise – A History of Opium", Macmillan, London 2018
2. McGreal C: "American Overdose – the Opioid Tragedy in Three Acts", Guardian Faber, London 2018
3. Paracelsus https://en.wikipedia.org/wiki/Paracelsus. Accessed on 5 June 2019
4. Inglis I: "Milk of Paradise – A History of Opium", Macmillan, London pps.69, 125,133,154-5,162,163-202, 202, 210, 214-19; 2018
5. Friedrich Sertürner. http://en.wikipedia.org/wiki/Friedrich_Sertürner. Accessed 9 June 2019
6. Kane H.H. The Hypodermic Injection of Morphia - its history, advantages and dangers. https://www.worldcat.org/title/hypodermic-injection-of-morphia-its-history-advantages-and-dangers/oclc/970765263. Accessed 9 June 2019
7. https://en.wikipedia.org/wiki/Harrison_Narcotics_Tax_Act. Accessed 12 June 2019
8. Mrs Winslow's Soothing Syrup. https://en.wikipedia.org/wiki/Mrs._Winslow%27s_Soothing_Syrup. Accessed on 7 June 2019

9. The Opium Trade with China. https://api.parliament.uk/historic-hansard/commons/1889/may/03/the-opium-trade-with-china. Accessed 7 June 2019.
10. Rushton S. https://www.bl.uk/romantics-and-victorians/articles/representations-of-drugs-in-19th-century-literature#. Accessed 12 June 2019
11. Castelow C https://www.historic-uk.com/HistoryUK/HistoryofBritain/Opium-in-Victorian-Britain/, Accessed 12 June 2019
12. BMA Board of Science, Drugs of dependence: the role of medical professionals. BMA; London, 2018 pp.87-88, 90, 91.
13. Johnson K, Gerada C, Greenhough A (2003) Treatment of neonatal abstinence syndrome. Archives of Disease in Childhood - Fetal and Neonatal Edition 2003;88:F2-F5.
14. Oliver A. 2019. Personal communication
15. Twycross R. Patient Care: Past, Present and Future. OMEGA 2007; 56: 7-19, 2007-2008
16. McGreal C: "American Overdose – the Opioid Tragedy in Three Acts", Guardian Faber, London 2018 pp. xiii, xiv, 21, 22, 23
17. ibid pp 293 - 298.
18. http://www.hhs.gov/opioids/ September 2018 accessed on 1 October 2019
19. https://www.nytimes.com/2016/05/07/opinion/the-opioid-epidemic-we-failed-to-foresee.html accessed on 1 October 2019
20. https://www.ons.gov.uk accessed on 1 October 2019
21. The Times September 28, 2019
22. https://www.rcoa.ac.uk/faculty-of-pain-medicine/opioids-aware/clinical-use-of-opioids/effectiveness-for-long-term-pain accessed on 1 October 2019
23. Knaul FM, Farmer PE et al (2018) Alleviating the access abyss in palliative care and pain relief—an imperative of universal health coverage: the Lancet Commission report. Lancet 391 pp 1331-1454
24. https://www.hrw.org/news/2017/10/12/report-lancet-calls-needed-pain-relief accessed on 1 October 2019.

Swaddling the Newborn Infant: Then and Now

PETER M. DUNN,
MA, MD, FRCP, FRCOG, FRCPCH
Emeritus professor of perinatal medicine and child health,
University of Bristol, UK. e-mail: P.M.Dunn@bristol.ac.uk

"And this shall be a sign to you; ye shall find the babe wrapped in swaddling clothes lying in a manger."
St. Luke's Gospel, 11, 6-7

1. Then

The custom of swaddling an infant during the first months of its life was both ancient and widespread, especially in cooler climates. It consisted of compressing the infant's body into a mummy-like mould using a system of tight bandages (Fig 1).

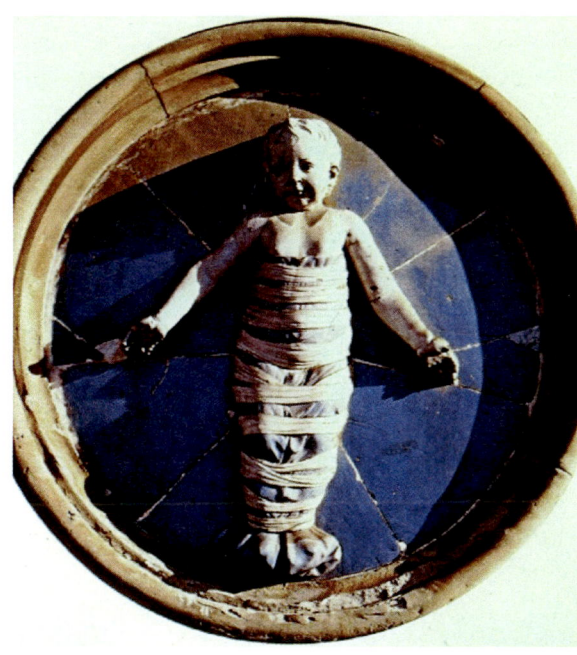

*Fig 1:
Swaddled infant
Andrea della Robia
(1435-1525), Florence*

Soranus of Ephesus (AD 98-138)[1] gave a detailed description of the practice, mentioning the orthopaedic reasons for swaddling in the following passage:

"Rather one must mould every part according to its natural shape, (and) if something has been

twisted during the time of delivery, one must correct it and bring it into its natural shape."

Galen (AD 129-200)[2] made similar recommendations adding that swaddling helped to protect the delicate skin of the newborn baby. He wrote:

"But when the baby is born, it is necessarily going to come in contact with cold and heat and with many bodies harder than itself. Therefore it is appropriate that his natural covering should be best prepared by us for exposure."

And he also added a warning:

"In little children ... their cries and screams ... mean something is annoying them ... It may be that they want warmth when they are cold, or cool when they are hot, or they are in discomfort from their swaddling bands, for even those are a burden ... I have also noticed that his cot and all his wrappings were too dirty and the infant himself dirty and unwashed, and I have ordered him to be bathed and that she should change his napkins for clean ones, and when these things were done the infant has stopped kicking and has settled off in a long sleep."

Some 1300 years later a book on children by Paulus Bagellardus gave almost identical instructions to those of Soranus on how to swaddle an infant (see Appendix[3]) and the practice remained popular in Europe until well into the 18th century (Fig 2).

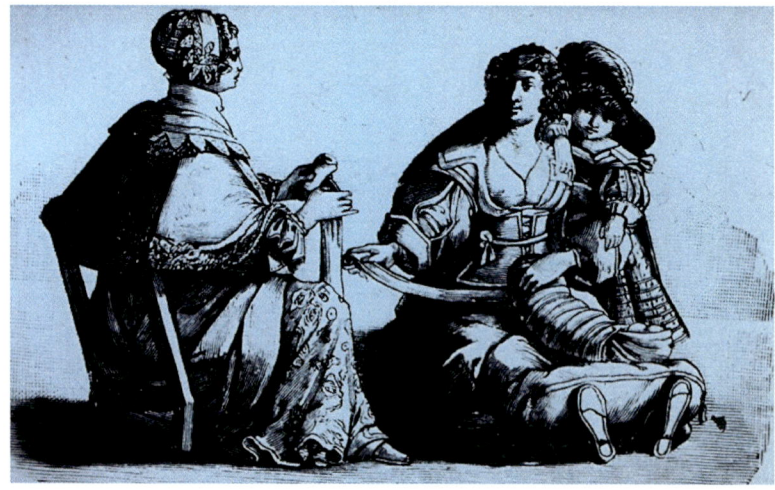

Fig 2: Women swaddling an infant (17thc)

Francois Mauriceau (1637-1709)[4], the famous French accoucheur, again recommended that: *"To prevent a child's growing crooked or awry or lame, the nurse must swaddle its body in a straight situation, equally extending the arms and legs."*

However, he added that:

"While all other animals have their bodies free, without the trouble of coverings, so they easily discharge themselves of their excretements ... it is not the same with infants who (being bound and swath'd with swathes and blankets, as we are forced, to give them a straight figure only suitable for mankind) cannot render their excretements."

Felix Würtz of Basel (1515-1575) was the first to sound a serious warning against swaddling. In his book on children[5] (1563) he wrote:

"I have seen children born straight, yet became lame and crooked, and could not be healed straight again; their mothers or nurses ... will not leave the birth as God hath created it, will have their children yet handsomer, by binding them straighter to their thinking, tye and bind them more crooked, doing it so hard, which maketh the child unquiet ... when children are bound straight with strong binding then they usually grow crooked; and none will grow more straight in his body, than those which are laid free and loose with their hands and feet: Therefore my advice is, not to use any curiousities at the laying and binding your children ..."

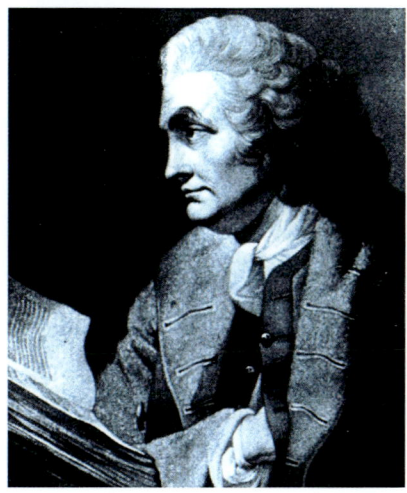

Fig 3: William Cadogan of Bristol (1711-1797)

John Locke (1632-1704) the English philosopher, also rejected swaddling in his book *'Some thoughts concerning education'* (1693) but it was Dr. William Cadogan of Bristol (1711-1797) (Fig 3) in his *'Essay upon the nursing and management of children from their birth to three years of age'* (1748)[6] who made the strongest plea for the universal abandonment of swaddling.

"Besides the mischief arising from the weight and heat of these swaddling-cloathes, they are put on so tight, and the child is so cramped by them, that its bowels have not room, nor the limbs any liberty, to act and exert themselves in the free easy manner they ought. This is a very hurtful circumstance; for limbs that are not used will never by strong, and such tender bodies cannot bear much pressure: the circulation restrained by the compression of any one part, just produce unnatural swellings in some other; especially as the fibres of infants are so easily distended. To which doubtless are owing the many distortions and deformities we meet with everywhere ..."

William Smellie (1697-1763)[7], the British man-midwife, also made an important observation in 1752 on the impact of tight binding on the respiration of an infant:

"I have been called several times, where I found the uneasiness of the children proceeded from too tight dressings; and by observing this circumstance in time, the danger was prevented by dressing them looser ... About two years ago, I was called to see a child, on the fourth day after delivery, and was told that it heaved, and had an oppression at its breast. The nurse undressed the child; and the clothes did not seem tight, but I observed the bandage on the navel appeared very tight. This I ordered to be unrolled; and plainly perceived that it was the cause of the disorder; for the child immediately breathed with greater freedom, and did very well in the sequel."

Jean Jacques Rousseau, the philospher of Geneva (1712-1778) wrote in 1762[8]:

"The child had hardly left the mother's womb, it had hardly begun to move and stretch its limbs, when it is given new bonds. It is wrapped in swaddling bands, laid down with its head fixed, its legs stretched out, and its arms by its side; it is wound round with linen and bandages of all sorts so that it cannot move ... Whence comes this unreasonable custom? ... A child unswaddled would need constant watching; well swaddled it is cast into a corner and its cries are ignored ... (Fig 4). It is claimed that infants left free would assume faulty positions and make movements which might injure the proper development of their limbs. This is one of the vain rationalizations of our false wisdom which experience has never confirmed."

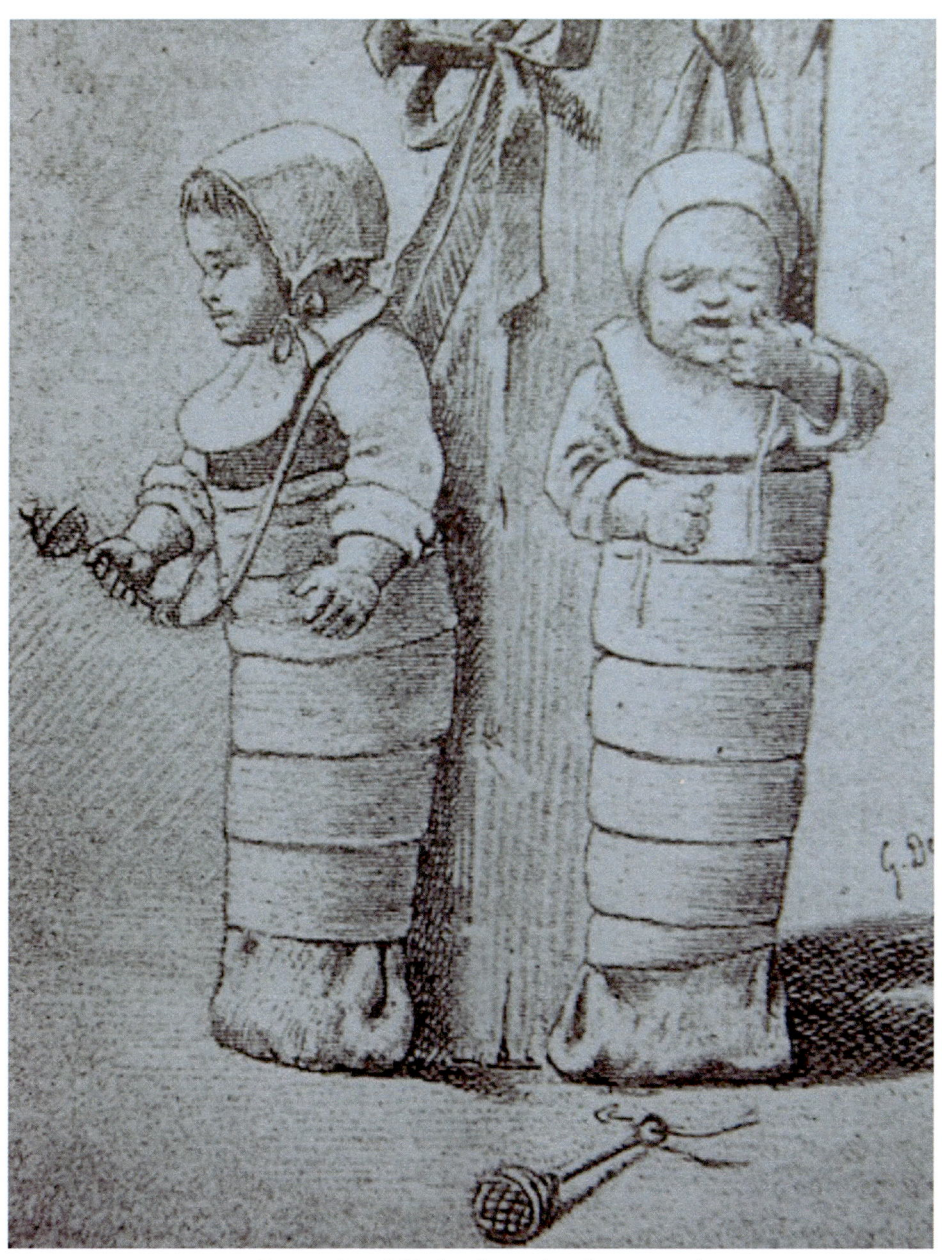

Fig 4: Swaddled infants (17th century)

Dr. William Heberden (1710-1801), a distinguished English physician, added his voice to the criticism of swaddling:

"Let them take example from nature and follow in her steps."

The great Swedish paediatrician, Nils Rosen, added his authority to the criticism of swaddling, writing in 1776[9]:

"The most approved practice would be never to swaddle children, which physicians have demonstrated by convincing arguments ... was a full grown person obliged to be thus swaddled, would he not think it a great hardship? But we seem to have no compassion on our innocent children."

How correct was Rosen in his assessment. It is distressing even to contemplate the suffering of infants in their tight swaddling, unable to move and exercise, to control their temperature, to breathe easily especially after feeds, and lying excoriating in their excreta often for long periods. Apart from the suffering, there can be little doubt that swaddling made a major contribution to the very high infant mortality of those early days (Fig 5).

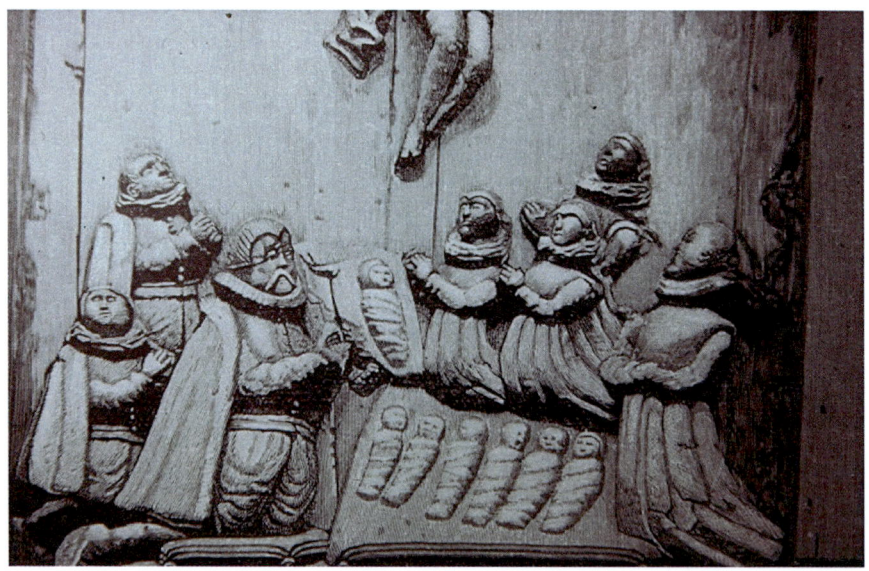

Fig 5: Family church memorial with seven swaddled newborn infants (1600)

As William Cadogan also wrote[6]:

"The mother who has only a few rags to cover her child loosely, and little more than her own breast to feed it, sees it healthy and strong, and very soon able to shift for itself: while the puny infant, the heir and hope of a rich family, lies languishing under a loan of finery that overpowers his limbs, abhorring and rejecting the dainties he is crammed with, till he dies a victim to the mistaken care and tenderness of his fond mother."

Gradually the practice of swaddling declined in Europe during the 17th and 18th centuries.

II. Now

Let us now fast forward 200 years to the second half of the 20th century. Swaddling in the UK seemed to have become a historical memory. However a vestigial remnant of it remained in the form of the umbilical binder. A crepe bandage around the abdomen was applied at birth with a view to protecting the umbilical stump from infection until it desiccated and fell off a few days later. In fact I discontinued the use of an umbilical binder in the maternity hospital where I was working as a registrar in 1960, as in my view it retarded desiccation and healing of the umbilical stump and encouraged infection. Furthermore, and more importantly, Professor John Emery (who had trained in Bristol) reported in 1967 two neonatal deaths that he attributed to tight umbilical binders [10] that, following a feed, had led to upward displacement of the diaphragm and obstructed respiration. This was the same problem previously described by William Smellie, the British man-midwife in 1752 [7]. Yet umbilical binders still continue to be used around the world.

Back in 1959 I commenced a ten year study on the aetiology of congenital postural deformities and in particular congenital dislocation of the hip (CDH). It led to my MD Thesis at Cambridge University[11]. I was able to show that quite gentle pressure, when maintained on the rapidly growing fetal hip joint, especially if the thighs were persistently adducted as in this case of frank breech presentation (Fig 6), might lead to dislocation. [12-14] I was also able to show that some 2% of

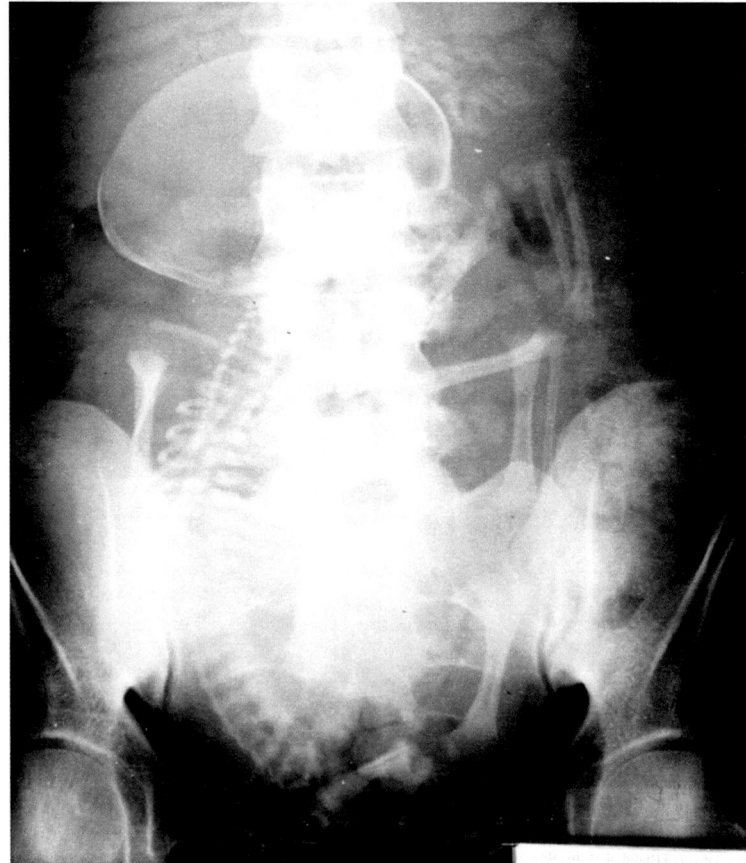

Fig 6: Frank breech presentation with legs flexed and adducted

newborn infants in the UK had unstable or dislocated hips at birth (Fig 7) though many of the dislocatable hips would stabilise in the days or weeks following delivery.

As a result, prior to the institution of neonatal screening and early treatment, the incidence for CDH at 2-3 years of age in Britain was around 1%, or around 7,000 new cases each year.

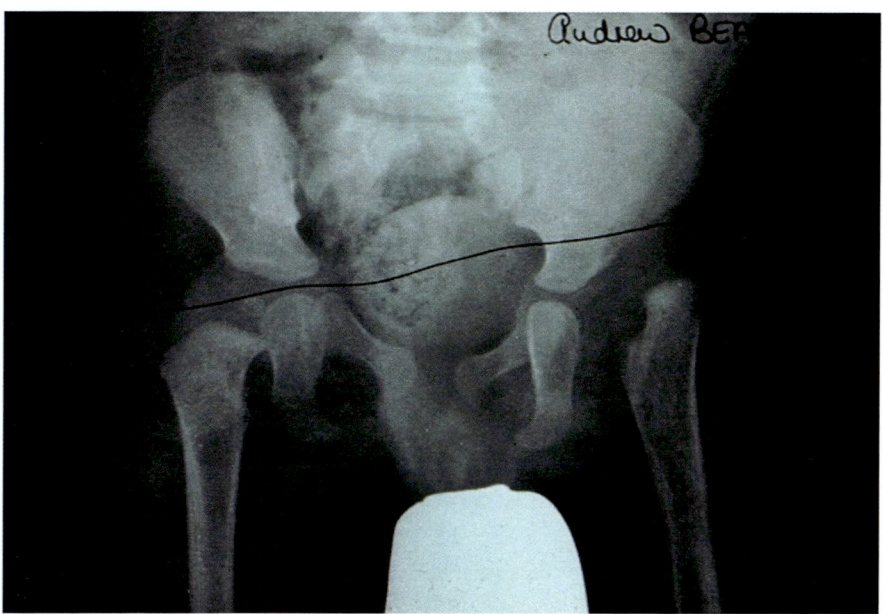

Fig 7: Congenital dislocation of the left hip at the age of 6 months

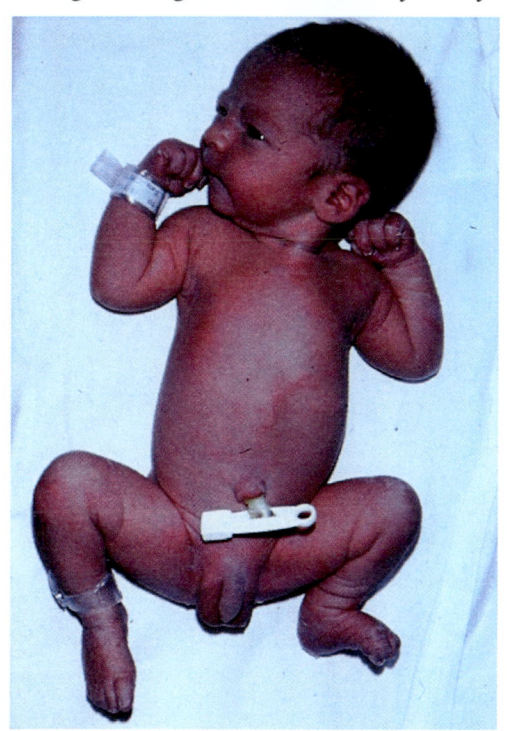

Fig 8: Newborn infant laying with thighs flexed and abducted

Newborn infants, when unconstrained, adopt a posture after birth with the hips flexed and abducted away from the line of the body (Fig 8). This is, in fact, the posture we use to treat infants diagnosed with CDH at birth (Fig 9).

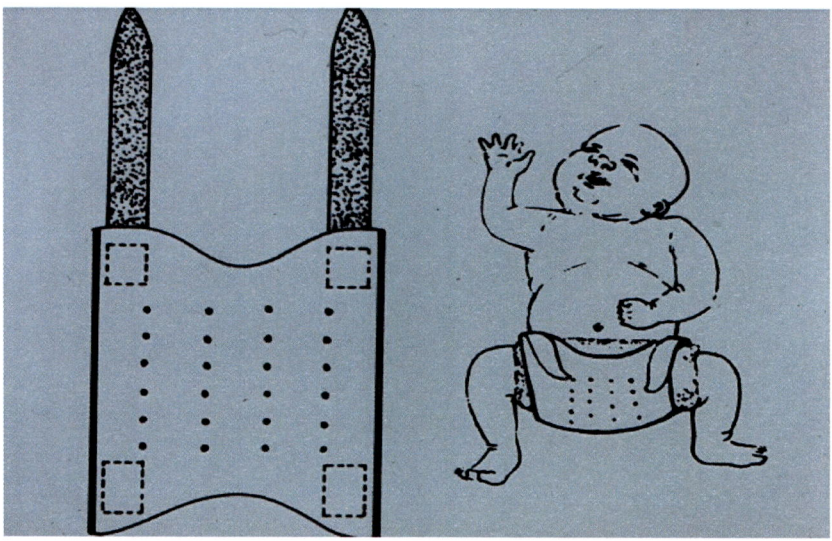

Fig 9: Aberdeen splint used for treating congenital dislocation of the hip

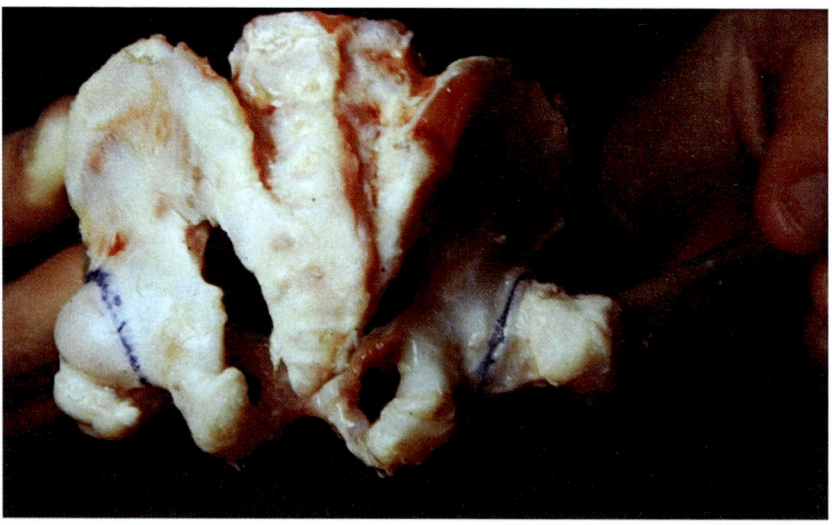

Fig 10: Posterior view of infant pelvis at postmortem: the left thigh is adducted and the right abducted. Note the exposure of the left head of femur outside the acetabulum

Abduction of the hip drives the head of the femur, through the anchor of the Y shaped ligament of the Bigalow, deep into the acetabulum, as in the abducted right thigh in this dissection seen from behind (see below). On the other hand, the thigh on the left is in adduction and much of the head of the femur is exposed and vulnerable to dislocation[15] (Fig 10).

Early in my study of the aetiology of CDH [11] I had become interested in the great variation in the incidence of this condition around the world. It was clear that while CDH was rare in many tropical countries, the incidence rose progressively as one moved into colder climates, reaching an incidence as high as 5-6% in the extreme north among the Lapplanders.

Since 1959 I have studied the way newborn infants are nursed by their mothers or carers. At first my knowledge was derived from the study of countless copies of the National Geographic magazine but later on by personally visiting some 80 countries around the world and seeing for myself. I now have an extensive collection of photos on how babies are nursed but will confine myself to showing just four. First, a baby in Swaziland nursed across his mother's back with his legs abducted (Fig 11). In South Africa, CDH is extremely rare.

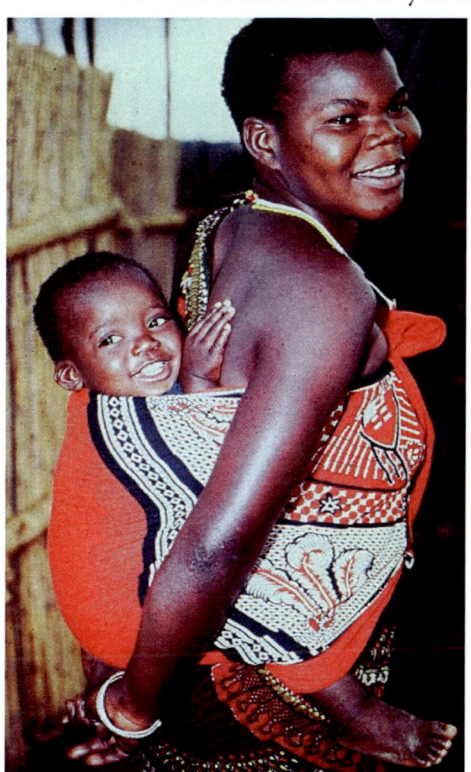

Fig 11: Swaziland lady carrying her infant with legs abducted

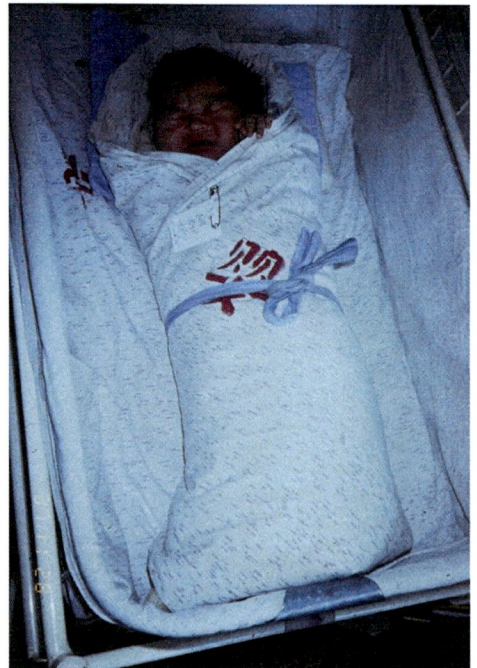

Second, an infant tightly wrapped in blankets in China (Fig 12). Thirdly, an infant even more tightly wrapped in Outer Mongolia (Fig 13) and finally a Red Indian baby in northern Canada in a papoose – a birch bark cradle permitting ready mobility in a hunter-gatherer society (Fig 14). The last three infants shown have their legs inevitably extended and adducted at the hip. Such populations have a high incidence of CDH.

Fig 12: (above) Chinese infant tightly wrapped (1987)

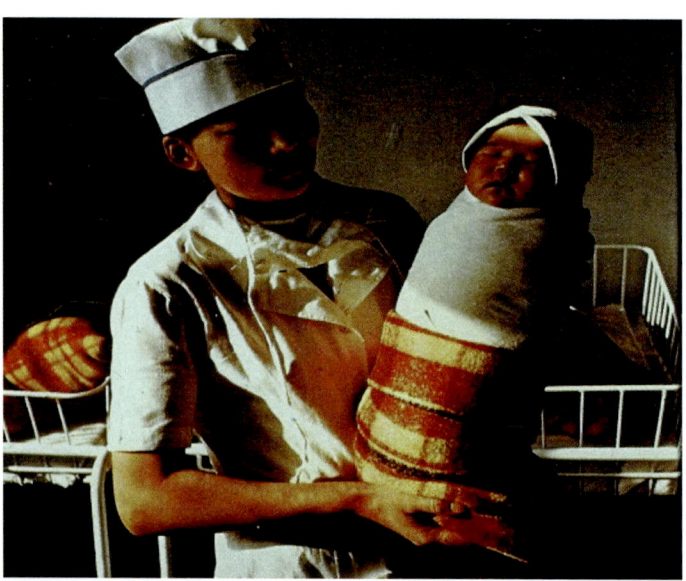

Fig 13: (Left) Swaddled infant in Outer Mongolia

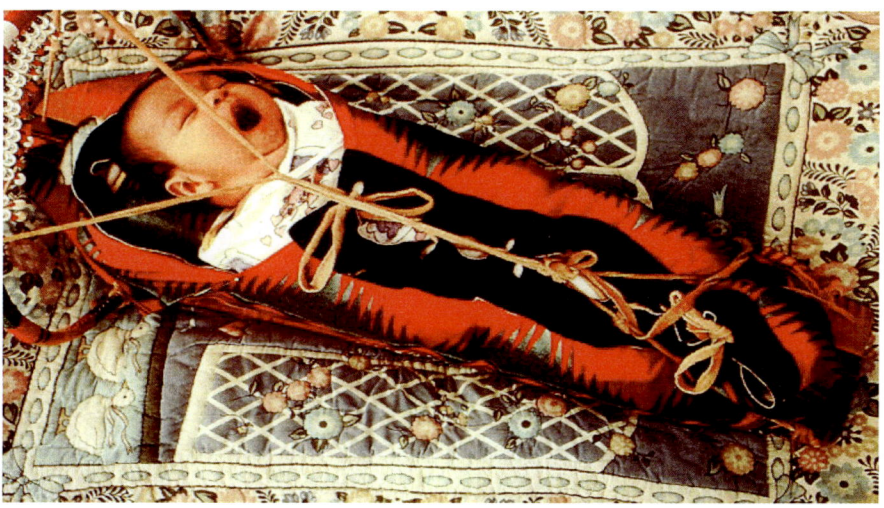

Fig 14: Red Indian baby in a papoose

Another factor appearing to influence the incidence of CDH is the season of birth. Reports from many countries including our own have noted an increase in the incidence of CDH, often a doubling, among infants born in the winter months. It has been suggested the colder weather leads to the use of heavier clothing and blankets which in turn restrict the infant's free movement and favour adduction of the thighs especially when the infant is lying on its side [11].

It is of interest that *de novo* infantile dislocation of the hip may occur as a complication of infants with congenital spastic diplegia (Little's disease) in which muscle spasm holds and maintains the legs in extension and tight adduction. This again lends support to the observation that the hip joint is vulnerable to dislocation when the legs are held persistently in adduction.

Nor is it just in remote lands that there is still a problem with swaddling. In many countries including our own, birthing now mainly takes place in hospital. Often for a variety of reasons, many of which are bad, babies are nursed separately from their mothers, only being united at intervals for feeding. To ease transfer the babies are often firmly wrapped in blankets. This is known as 'bundling' but is not that different from swaddling on its effect on the infant.

Since the 1990s some doctors have promoted swaddling suggesting that not only do infants sleep better and cry less [16], but that this method of nursing may protect them against cot deaths. However, research undertaken by Professor Peter Fleming and his colleagues here in the south west has shown that swaddling may actually significantly increase the risk of the sudden infant death syndrome [17,18].

In my view, swaddling (and its counterpart, bundling) is a practice in modern infant care that should be abandoned forthwith. Not only does it increase the incidence of that most common crippling deformity, congenital dislocation of the hip, which in later life may cause most painful arthritis but it may also lead to *de novo* infantile dislocation of the hip. It also prevents the infant from exercising its muscles and joints. Swaddling may also rob the infant of its ability to control its temperature. Hyperthermia, as well as hypothermia, may prove fatal [19]. In addition, swaddling, especially after feeds, may embarrass respiration. Alternatively it may lead to regurgitation, inhalation and pulmonary infection. Furthermore it is possible that it may be responsible for later psychological problems. This is fertile ground for further research. Luckily our memories are not good in the first year of life but which of us as adults would survive without psychological damage if we were severely constrained in a way not dissimilar to the use of a straight jacket for a period of several months.

I repeat, swaddling should be universally discarded as a most undesirable and dangerous practice.

Appendix

Bagellardus, P. (1472)
Libellus de egritudinibus infantium.
Cited by Ruhräh, J. In: Pediatrics of the past. New York, 1925, p.34
Swaddling
'After this, she should cover the infant's head with a fine linen cloth after the manner of a hood. Then secure a soft linen cloth and with the infant placed on the midwife's lap in such a way that its head is toward her feet and its feet rest upon her body, the midwife should roll it in the linen cloth, after it has been bathed, wrapping its feet. First with its arms

raised above, she should warp its breast and bind its body with a band, by three or four windings. Next the midwife takes another piece of linen or little cloth and draws the hands of the infant straight forward towards the knees and hips, shaping them evenly, so that the infant acquires no humpiness. She then, with the same assisting band, binds and wraps the infant's arms and hands, all of which will be correctly shaped. Then she should turn the infant over on its breast with its back raised upward and, taking hold of the infant's feet, make its soles touch its buttocks to the end that its knees might be properly set. Thereupon she should straighten the infant's legs and with another band and little cloths bind and wrap up the hips. Next take the entire infant and roll it in a woollen cloth or after our manner in a cape lined with sheep skins; and this in winter, but in summer a linen cloth simply.'

References

1. Soranus. Gynecology. Transl. by O. Tempkin. Baltimore, Johns Hopkins Press, 1956.
2. Dunn, P.M. Galen (AD129-200) of Pergamun: anatomist and experimental physiologist. Arch. Dis. Child. Fetal Neonatal Ed. 2003; 88, F441-F443.
3. Bagellardus, P. Libellus de egritudinibus infantium, 1472.
4. Mauriceau, F. Diseases of women with child and in childbed. Transl. by H. Chamberlen, London, 8th edition, 1752.
5. Würtz, F. The Children's Book of Felix Würtz, 1656.
6. Dunn, P.M. Dr. William Cadogan (1711-1797) of Bristol and the management of infants. Arch. Dis. Childh., 1992; 67, 72-73.
7. Dunn, P.M. Dr. William Smellie (1697-1763), the master of British midwifery. Arch. Dis. Childh., 1995; 72, F77-F78.
8. Rousseau, J-J. Emile: or on education, 1762.
9. Dunn, P.M. Dr. Nils Rosen (1706-1773): the father of paediatrics in Sweden. Arch. Dis. Childh., 1991; 66, 1171-1172.
10. Emery, J.L. Tight umbilical binders. Proc. Roy. Soc. Med., 1967; 60, 49-50.
11. Dunn, P.M. The influence of the intrauterine environment in the causation of congenital postural deformities, with special reference to congenital dislocation of the hip. MD thesis, Cambridge University, 1969.

12. Dunn, P.M. Perinatal observations on the aetiology of congenital dislocation of the hip. Clin. Orthop., 1976; 119, 11-22.
13. Dunn, P.M., Evans, R.E., Thearle, M.J., Griffiths, H.E.D. and Witherow, P.J. Congenital dislocation of the hip: early and late diagnosis and management compared. Arch. Dis. Childh., 1985; 60, 407-414.
14. Dunn, P.M. Pitfalls in the early diagnosis of congenital dislocation of the hip. West Engl. Med. J., 2017 (June), 116, 1-5.
15. Dunn, P.M. The anatomy and pathology of congenital dislocation of the hip. Clin. Orthop., 1976; 119, 23-27.
16. Franco, P., Seret, N., van Hees, J.N, Scaillet, S., Grosswasser, J. and Kahn, A. Influence of swaddling on sleep and arousal characteristics of healthy infants. Pediatrics, 2005; 115, 1307-11.
17. Blair, PS., Sidebotham, P., Evason-Coombe, C., Edmonds, M., Heckstall, E.M., Fleming, P. Hazardous co-sleeping environments and risk factors amenable to change: case control study of SIDS in south west England. Brit. Med., J., 2009; 339, 3666.
18. Pease, A.S., Fleming, P.J., Hanck, F.R., Moon, R.Y., Horne, R.S.C., L'Hoir, M.P., Ponsonby, A-L. and Blair, P.S. Swaddling and the risk of Sudden Infant Death Syndrome: a meta-analysis. Pediatrics, 2016; 137, e20153275.
19. Cheng, T.L., Partridge, J.C. Effect of binding and high environmental temperature on neonatal body temperature. Pediatrics, 1993; 92, 238-240.

Scottish Doctors in the Imperial Russian Court

BRUNO BUBNA-KASTELIZ
Presented at the meeting on June 3rd 2019

Scottish doctors seem to have been pre-eminent in their profession in 18th century Britain, most of them having studied in one of the three Scottish medical schools at the time – Aberdeen, Glasgow or Edinburgh. Certainly many Scottish medical alumni practised all over Europe and travelled more widely than other UK graduates. The famous medical centres in Europe – Padua, Leyden or Vienna were still producing very skilled and innovative graduates - but it was Scottish medical graduates who were often invited to practise in the courts of Europe.

I shall discuss three Scottish doctors who served successively as private physicians to the Imperial Court of Russia between 1768 and 1840 - Drs. Dimsdale, Rogerson and Wylie. There were many other Scottish doctors who also practised in Russia, some of them attaining Court Physician status, others gaining high positions in the Russian Army Medical Corps. Among them were Drs. Robert Erskine (Peter the Great, i.e. early 1700s), Matthew Guthrie (Imperial Russian Army, 1760s), James Grieve (Empress Elizabeth), his son John Grieve, James Mounsey, who married James Grieve's daughter and was an uncle of Rogerson and finally Sir Alexander Crichton. I won't have the time to talk about that second group in the present session.

Dr. Thomas Dimsdale (1712–1800)

The Dimsdale family was a dynasty of doctors who had settled in Hertfordshire in the mid-17th century and were Quakers. There was at least one Dr. Dimsdale, and at one time even three at the same time, recorded in Bishops Stortford over the whole 18th and 19th centuries. One of them, however, Thomas Dimsdale (figure 1) son of Dr. William Dimsdale, was a holder of a medical degree from Aberdeen and was to become the most famous member of the family for two reasons. He was one of the earliest pioneers of inoculation for smallpox and went on to be invited to St. Petersburg to be personal physician to the then Empress of Russia, Catherine the Great.

Thomas Dimsdale published this pamphlet in 1767 (figure 2).

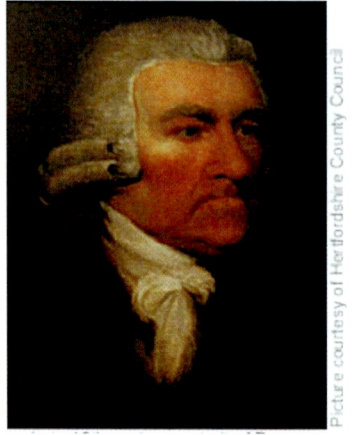

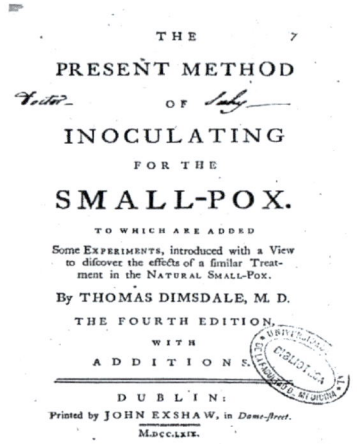

Figure 1.
Late 18th century portrait of
Baron Thomas Dimsdale MD

Figure 2
The 1769, 4th edition of his paper on
smallpox inoculation

Smallpox was considered to be an exceptionally serious disease, so much so that in Bishop's Stortford an apothecary was appointed to provide all the medicines necessary for inmates of the workhouse, except in the case of smallpox. All persons infected by smallpox, however, were isolated in the 'Pest House' that stood at the top of Maze Green Road. Thomas Dimsdale's method was to inoculate a healthy patient using matter from someone who already had the disease. The patient would then suffer an attack of smallpox, but due to adequate preparations was able to recover quickly and so become immune to further infection. He also advocated a strict regime of diet, fresh air and gentle exercise both before and after inoculation. It was naturally a far more hazardous undertaking than vaccination as we know it today, which follows the Edward Jenner (1749–1823) method first used in 1796. The latter's initial experiments, if you remember, involved inoculation with the related cow-pox virus to build immunity against the deadly smallpox virus. Originally, probably in the 15th century, the Chinese had been using the inhalation of scabs from infected people's variola pustules, which of course had very variable results, many leading to severe infection and death and only a small number of inoculants surviving a milder form of the disease. After at least 300 years this form of variolation eventually reached the Ottoman Empire, where the wife of the British Ambassador to

Constantinople, Lady Mary Wortley-Montgue, came across it in the early years of the 18th century and it was gradually taken up in Europe. Dimsdale's technique involved the use of a fine, sterile silk thread, which was drawn through the infectious pustules of a carefully chosen individual and then sealed in small glass vials. A new vial was selected for each recipient, and after scratching their forearms the thread from the vial was drawn through the fresh wound. Those subject to variolation were then quarantined, in just the same way as natural smallpox cases until the mild and localized infection had come and gone (typically a three to four week period).

In October of the year following the first publication of his paper, i.e. 1768, Thomas was invited to the far-off court of Catherine the Great, Empress of Russia. At that time, outbreaks of smallpox were devastating populations worldwide. Russia was said to have a mortality rate of about an 80%. So to safeguard her people, and set an example, the Empress volunteered to be immunised herself. Thomas Dimsdale and his son, Nathaniel, made the journey to St Petersberg with enough vials to inoculate the entire court. For Dimsdale's part, he insisted that he should test the process on the courtiers before the Empress herself. Catherine refused this and instructed him to treat her first, and then following a successful outcome, to treat her son. The dubious safety record of variolation is underlined by the precautions both Dimsdale and his royal host had to undertake. Had anything gone wrong, it is said Catherine ordered horses to be kept at regular intervals from St Petersburg to Holland to whisk the doctor away should the Russians seek vengeance against him and his son. Thankfully all went well, and the grateful Catherine showered the doctor with gifts of diamonds and furs, plus £12,000 and an annuity of £500 (respectively worth well over £10 million and £400,000 annually today). He was also bestowed with a hereditary barony of the Russian Empire, which is still held by the family and the first to have been conferred in Russia.

Thomas married as his third wife, his cousin Elizabeth, great grand-daughter of Robert Dimsdale. They married in 1780 and in 1781 she accompanied her now internationally renowned husband back to Russia. The tsarina had invited him back to inoculate her youngest son, Crown Prince Alexander. They sailed from Dover in the June, returning at the end of November the same year. Elizabeth kept a journal of their travels and her observations while in Russia, all of which provide a very valuable snapshot of the period from the rare perspective of a woman and which was later published. Thomas later sat as an MP for Hertford in two parliaments in 1780 and 1784, before his death in 1800 at the age of 88. He requested to be buried in the Friends' burial ground in Bishops Stortford, now a small private garden.

*****

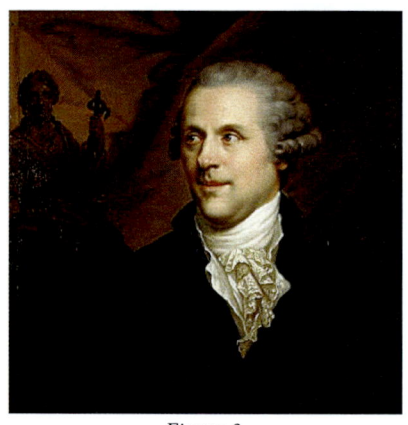

Figure 3
Dr. John Samuel Rogerson (1740-1828)

John Rogerson (figure 3) was born to Samuel Rogerson and his wife Janet Johnston, in lower Annandale (Lochbrow) on 22 October 1740. His life began in a small tenant farm and ended eighty-four years later in Dumcrieff House less than five miles from where it began. His affinity for Scotland remained throughout his life and recognition of his achievements in his profession was accorded upon his return when he was made a freeman of Dumfries. As a teenager, he was a frequent and welcome visitor to the Clerk family who had acquired Dumcrieff House, near Moffatt, as their summer house. He was observing their efforts to improve the property, add more rooms to it and generally improve its interior and in the grounds, to repair fencing and dyking and to create a plantation of forest trees. John must have been saddened when his good friend, George Clerk had to close his linen factory in Dumfries and sell Dumcrieff House in 1782.

At home, the news from Russia was that John Rogerson's uncle James Mounsey was doing very well now practising there as a doctor. Mounsey had availed himself of the opportunity to attend lectures at Paris University and eventually while in Paris emerged with a medical qualification. After five years with the Navy, he opted for private practice in Saint Petersburg where he remained and was eventually appointed as private doctor to the obese Empress Elizabeth. After her death, her son Peter III awarded Dr Mounsey the rank of Privy Councillor. Because he was increasingly unpopular for waging wars with neighbours Peter III was assassinated only six months after becoming Tsar. He was replaced by his wife Catherine II, a member of the German aristocracy and who was to gain glory later as Catherine the Great. Mounsey retired and returned to Scotland wealthy and built himself the luxurious mansion of Rammerscales, near Hightae, Dumfries and Galloway.

Mounsey's return gave John Rogerson, by then a medical student in Edinburgh, the chance to discuss with his uncle in great detail the situation and prospects in Russia. He was encouraged to seek a career there. Soon after obtaining his medical degree in 1765, he too left for St. Petersburg via Elsinore in Denmark, arriving in the Russian capital some time in 1766. On 5 September 1766 he was interviewed by a three member Committee and gained his permit to practice medicine in Russia. Following that, an Imperial "ukaz" (Governmental decree) appointed him as "Court Doctor" in February 1769. His next task was to learn Russian. He quite easily learned to speak it, but his writing of it was always bad. However, he won respect and widespread sympathy among the nobility of St Petersburg.

He paid several visits to Scotland from his post in St. Petersburg. Two of the visits were connected to formal occasions: in 1782 he became a member of the Royal College of Physicians of Edinburgh. Four years later he was to receive the Freedom of the City of Dumfries. Other, unrecorded, visits were to see his father and relatives, but also to look for farm properties to buy. The aim was not to derive personal gain - which he did not need. Rather, he wished to provide opportunities for his son and *"to make a difference"*, like his father, to the lives of as many of his tenant farmers as possible. The first recorded purchase by Rogerson was of the Gillesbie Estate in 1782. The most expensive was the large Wamphray estate which cost him £90,000, a very large sum in 1810 (probably as much as £5M today). But it was in 1805 that he bought Dumcrieff House. Rogerson must have seen the chance to secure for his retirement a wealth of happy memories.

There is a delightful anecdote of him in St. Petersburg, described by an English visitor in his Travels. 'Dr. Rogerson,' he says, 'as *we were informed, regularly received*' (from his patients' hands) '*his snuff-box, and as regularly carried it to a jeweller for sale. The jeweller sold it again to the first Russian nobleman who wanted a fee for his physician; so that the doctor obtained his box again, and at last the matter became so well understood between the jeweller and the physician, that it was considered by both parties as a sort of banknote, and no words were necessary in transacting the sale of it.*' These 'bank notes' allowed Dr. Rogerson to become rich enough to acquire the estate of Wamphray, in his native Dumfriesshire. It was the same traveller who also wrote that *'Persons calling themselves English Physicians are found in almost every town in Russia.'*

In 1819 Dr. Rogerson was already some 78 years old and was, at last, organising his departure from St. Petersburg. He entrusted his nephew Alexander, who was employed by the solicitors J. Thomson, T. Bonar & Co, with two tasks: the sale of his house and to take care of his serfs.

Dr. Rogerson did not need to take with him to Scotland the strong and much praised carriage that the renowned coach maker Alexander Crichton in Edinburgh had built for him on order and delivered in St Petersburg some years ago. He could just order another one locally.

Once back in Scotland, Dr. Rogerson did not take residence immediately in the mansion he had acquired some years before. He considered the building too small and unpretentious for a person of his wealth and status. He therefore decided to have it demolished and replaced on the same site with a new one of a size and on plans he would approve personally. Demolition and rebuilding would take time and Dr. Rogerson was staying in the meantime partly in Edinburgh but mostly in Moffat, at the residence of his friend, the Earl of Hopetoun (the present Moffat House Hotel). This enabled him to keep an eye on the work and ensure the result he envisaged. Only one room of the old building, an erstwhile dining room, was saved and incorporated in the new, as a reminder of the happy times of George Clerk's hospitality.

The building work at Dumcrieff progressed and Dr Rogerson was satisfied, as he announced to a friend on 28 March 1820: *"I am glad the work is going so well at Dumcrieff and I should think that it will be right to have the additional offices erected as early as may be"*. He was right, and a few weeks later he was at last in residence in the mansion of his dreams.

On 21 December 1823 Dr John Rogerson died at Dumcrieff and was buried on the 29th at the Wamphray Glen churchyard. There is now in that rural churchyard a simple roofless *"enclosure"* where a memorial plaque carries the bare inscription: *"In memory of Dr John Rogerson of Wamphray, First physician to His Majesty the Emperor of Russia born 1741, died 2 Dec 1823 at the age of 82 years"*.

****

James Wylie was born in Kincardine-on-Forth on 13th November 1768, the son of a carrier. Kinkardine was a busy seaport where at the time some 90 ships were registered. Eager to dive deep into life as a young man, James Wylie attempted to run away by sea only to be dragged from the docks back home by his mother. If it were not for her maternal instincts, he would never have had the opportunity to save hundreds of lives himself. The vessel he had planned to board sailed from Cramond and sank within a day during

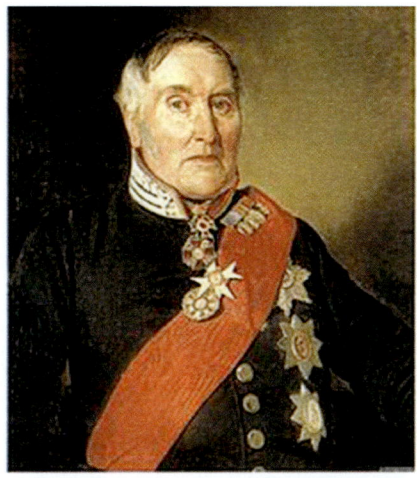

Figure 4. Sir James Wylie (1768-1854)

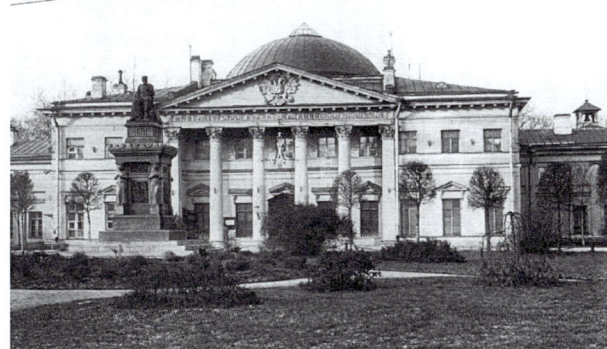

Figure 5. Wylie's Military Medical Academy, St. Petersburg

a violent storm. Wylie had escaped certain drowning.

He was initially apprenticed to a local doctor, Dr Meldrum but Wylie started attending the University of Edinburgh in 1786 and took classes in anatomy, surgery and medical theory & practice. There he learned his profession from great figures of the Scottish Enlightenment, such as Alexander Monro, Joseph Black and William Cullen. However, as was not uncommon at that time, he left without graduating after leaving home in mysterious circumstances ... believed to be linked to sheep stealing!

In 1790 Wylie left for St Petersburg. It is there that he was to spend the rest of his life in the service of the Russian people. He went on to become perhaps the most influential medical man in 19th century Russia. For twenty-five years he directed the Army Medical Department and was effectively the head of the whole profession. Figure 5 shows the Medico-Chirurgical Academy he founded. Wylie rose from regimental surgeon to become the personal doctor to three Russian Emperors, president of the Medico-Chirurgical Academy and Russia's only other baronet.

Shortly after his arrival in St. Petersburg in 1790, Wylie had joined the Eletsky Regiment and as Regimental Surgeon was present with his men at the Siege of Warsaw in 1794 and of Cracow in 1795. He then saved the life of the Danish Ambassador, Baron Otto von Bloom, where other surgeons including a Scottish one, had failed and in consequence Wylie was appointed to the Royal Household in 1795. He then devoted himself to medical research, producing a paper on yellow fever in Russian that earned him an MD from Aberdeen University. Subsequently, a dramatic life-saving operation made his reputation. Count Kutaisoff, one of the Empress's favourite courtiers, was in danger of suffocation from an abscess in his neck. His physicians, probably through professional jealousy, were slow to ask advice from Rogerson as the Court surgeon and it was only when the patient was on the point of death that Wylie was called in. Wylie did not hesitate, draining the abscess and saving Kutaisoff's life. It is thought he probably had performed the first tracheotomy in Russia. Years later, Wylie used to recount how he *"owed his promotion to cutting Count Kutaisov's throat"*. This episode attracted the interest of the heir to the Imperial throne Paul who in 1798 succeeded his mother Catherine and appointed Wylie his personal physician and surgeon with rooms in the Royal Palace. His service with this Tsar Paul I was to be short lived, for in 1801 the Tsar's mental state deteriorated rapidly, and he was strangled to death in St Michael's Castle by a group of drunken army officers. Wylie and two other Scottish doctors performed the post mortem examination and issued the death certificate declaring that Paul died of apoplexy. Wylie must therefore have been involved in that intrigue. It was a tactful and diplomatic action but nonetheless a deception that was only revealed as such to the Western world in 1907.

Wylie's career in the military service of the Tsars and of Russia was long and distinguished. Despite, or perhaps because of, his friendship with royalty Wylie continued on active military service. During the Napoleonic Wars he was present at the Battle of Austerlitz in 1805, Jena in 1806 and Borodino in 1812, a devasting battle in which the Russian army lost 45,000 men. It was at Borodino that Wylie surpassed himself, carrying out over 200 operations on the battlefield, many of them amputations. It is thought that it is Wylie to whom Tolstoy refers in his description of a surgeon in the battle in his War and Peace. Not only did Wylie perform heroic feats of surgery on the field of battle, but also on the night following Borodino he rode with the Cossacks under the command of Platoff deep into the French lines. In recognition of all this he was knighted and made Baronet of the United Kingdom in London in 1814 by the Prince Regent on a visit to England to be made a Fellow of the Royal College of Physicians of Edinburgh. In 1824 he himself was injured and such was his regard for Wylie that Czar Alexander sat at Wylie's bedside for three days. Wylie's admiration for the Cossacks is shown on his coat of arms which displays a Cossack on horseback at full speed holding a spear.

Wylie in turn cared for Tsar Alexander I. He had saved his life more than once but the Czar eventually died of Crimean Fever in 1825. Wylie attended Alexander I during his last illness and was one of those who signed the autopsy report. This loss of his friend affected Wylie greatly but the new Tsar Nicholas I continued Wylie's appointment as his personal physician. Though getting on for 60, he visited and inspected the hospitals personally to ensure that high standards were maintained. For 25 years he directed the Army Medical Department and was effectively the head of the whole profession. Wylie rose from regimental surgeon to become the personal doctor to four Russian Emperors (Paul I, Peter III, Alexander I and Nicholas I) and President of the Medico-Chirurgical Academy.

He was skilled as a physician as well as surgeon and used many of his own remedies, for instance *'Solution Mineralis'* to cure malaria. He continued to teach students even when he was the Tsar's personal physician. Wylie received many accolades and awards and many valuable gifts in recognition of his services. He continued to be active till late in life and he remained mentally alert and in good health till his death at the age of 85 in 1854 in St Petersburg. At the time of his death, he was a privy councillor, holding numerous Russian and foreign honours, as well as enjoying considerable personal wealth. Most of his estate was bequeathed to the Tsar and in St Petersburg a clinic was built and named after him. He was buried in the city in the presence of the Tsar and all the Court such was their regard for him. Wylie never married and he left his estate to the Russian nation for the construction of a large hospital for teaching the pupils of the Medico-Chirurgical Academy.

Sir James Wylie was one of the last and best-remembered pioneering medical Scots who worked in Russia during the early 19th century. The hospital where he worked, the clinic founded with his bequest and his statue still stand in St Petersburg today. The statue of him in the grounds of the Army Medical Academy was moved (see the statue in on figure 5) to the hospital which he founded. Now, thanks to the efforts of Kincardine Community Council, a plaque has been erected in his birthplace. The unveiling was carried out by Barbara Neish, a distant relative of Wylie, who travelled from her home in Bermuda to take part in the ceremony.

Scottish doctors and slavery.
MIKE DAVIDSON FRCS DHMSA

This talk is based on research for my M. Litt in Scottish Heritage dissertation at the University of Aberdeen. The dissertation uses the journals of Dr Jonathan Troup held in the Special Collections of the University of Aberdeen, comparing his observations and views on Dominican society and the illnesses he encounters. The journal covers the periods of Troups' journeys to and from Dominica, where he worked as a doctor treating both free and enslaved populations. The collection also includes his journals of his work as a country doctor in rural Aberdeenshire. Given the time limitations, it is perhaps best described as an introduction to medical practitioners' involvement in the slave-based economies of the British West Indies. I apologise in advance for any language or concepts regarding African slaves that I know will be unacceptable to modern ears, but they reflect the attitudes of some of our ancestors. In discussing Medicine and slavery, mention should be made not only of the Slave trade, i.e. the enforced transportation of African slaves, but also the slave plantation-based economies of the British colonies.

Until recently the involvement of Scots in the institution of slavery has received little academic interest. In an interview with Russell Leadbetter of the Sunday Herald in October 2015, Prof. T. Devine states *"For many years Scotland's historians harboured the illusion that our nation had little to do with the slave trade or plantation slavery."* Iain Whyte, author of Scotland and the Abolition of Slavery, speaking of Scots and slavery is quoted in the Daily Record in 2007 *"We swept it under the carpet. This was remarkable in the light of Glasgow's wealth coming from tobacco, sugar and cotton, and Jamaica Streets being found in several Scottish towns and cities."* Scotland can be considered to show a degree of national amnesia when considering its past involvement in slavery. Historians of Scotland's past have concentrated on the undoubted major contribution of Scots to the abolition movement. I would suggest a similar amnesia could apply to the study of the medical professions within the slave-based economies.

While the England and Scotland crowns had united under the Stuarts in 1603, the two nations did not integrate until the Act of Union in 1707. The Union was, in part, a result of the failed Scottish colony in Darien (1698 – 1700). Political and economic Union gave Scots increased access to the developing English colonies of North America and the West Indies. The predominance of Scottish medical training in the 18th century Britain and an overcrowded professional market in Scotland resulted in the emigration of Scottish trained doctors to the slave-based colonies. Recruitment of doctors was by the same networks of universities, advertising, medical societies we are familiar with today but also the networks of kinship and patronage for which the Scots were well known.

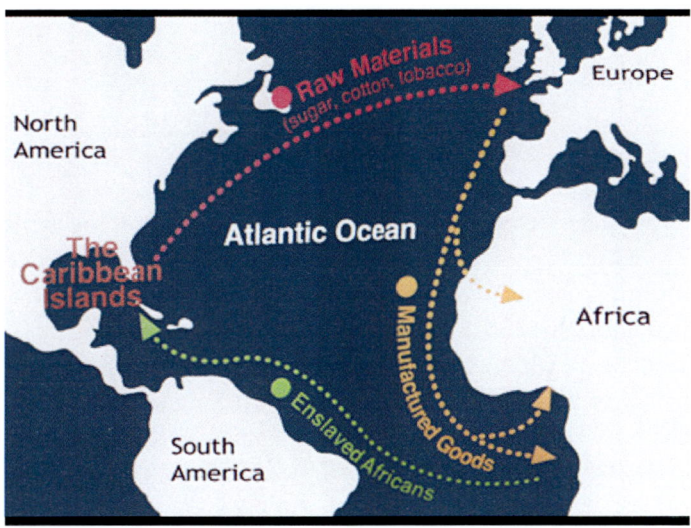

Triangular Slave trade 17th – early 19th century.

Slave Trade and doctors.

The Slave trade and plantation economy was a triangular transatlantic series of trade routes. Manufactured goods, alcohol, arms, metal work etc. were taken to West Africa and exchanged with local Kings or middle men for captives. Local wars were often aggravated by Europeans to increase the captive supply. The slaves were selected, inoculated against TB and held in coastal forts. The transatlantic transfer, the infamous "Middle Passage", was in overcrowded ships where the slave mortality was over 20%; the ships crews also had a 20% mortality. The surviving slaves were sold in the West Indies, often after being *"seasoned"* (exposed to indigenous fevers); the mortality rate reached as high as 33 percent in Jamaica.

Ships surgeons were valued as a means of maximising profits by reducing shipboard mortality. They medically screened and inoculated slaves on the African coast and attempted to maintain some degree of hygiene and sanitation on the ship, often treating slaves with stimulative and supportive medicines. Research shows that by the late 18th century 40% of the surgeons within the British slave trade were from Scotland at a time when Scots made up only 10% of Britain's population. Suzanne Schwarz, in her chapter in Prof. Devine's book *Recovering Scotland's slavery past*, gives details of the Liverpool slave trade doctors. It is very well referenced, comparing the activity of Scottish doctors who were abolitionists, often after witnessing slave ships first hand, and those who strongly supported the slave trade.

In 1788, William Dolben M.P., an abolitionist, supported a parliamentary act ordering all slave ships to carry a doctor who had to keep records about the enslaved Africans on board. The act also specified that the crew should be paid a bonus if less than 3% of the slaves died on the voyage. Conditions however remained appalling and it is debatable if there was major reduction in the mortality of crew or the enslaved following the Dolben Act.

Slave Ship doctors and those at the West Africa slave forts were known as guinea surgeons; often they were surgeon apothecaries with a military background. Here are two examples whose careers illustrate typical progression with the slave trade:

Archibald Dalzel 1740 – 1811 was born in Kirkliston in Scotland and trained to be a doctor in Edinburgh. In 1763, after a spell in the navy, he went to Africa as a slave fort surgeon but started trading slaves to add to his salary. After serving as a slave ship's surgeon, he captained several voyages. In 1764 he wrote *"I have come a little into the spirit of the slave trade and must own, perhaps it ought to be my shame, that I can now traffic in that way without remorse."* He went on to be a planter on the Mississippi but, after losses in the War of Independence, returned to slave ship captaincy.

James Irving Snr. (1731-1807) built a successful career in the slave trade of eighteenth-century Liverpool, firstly as a ship's surgeon and then as a captain. In line with Scottish kin networks, he supported his nephew James Irving's career as a ship's surgeon on the slave ships. Details of his life are covered in the book *Slave Captain - The Career of James Irving in the Liverpool Slave Trade* by Suzanne Schwarz.

Doctors in the British West Indies in the era of slavery.

Recruitment of medical practitioners to the Caribbean colonies in the late eighteenth century was needed to reduce the mortality of the military, the enslaved and white colonists. Following European colonisation, the West Indies could be considered a cauldron of diseases, a nexus of diseases from Europe and West Africa and indigenous ailments. Following the decline of the aboriginal population due to introduced disease, a continuing high mortality of recent arrivals meant a significant population flux.

Most Scots in the Caribbean planned to return with their wealth to Britain, i.e. sojourning. An example of a successful doctor, though I use the word doctor advisedly, was *Alexander Grant*. His story is not unusual. At 17, after studying basic pharmacy for a year in Aberdeen, he migrated to Jamaica. he worked as a doctor to the slaves on his cousin's sugar plantations. Within ten years he had bought his own plantation and opened a trading company in Kingston. In 1737 he married the daughter of a wealthy English plantation owner. They moved to London in 1739, where Grant expanded his business, including part ownership of a slave trading African fort. When he died in 1772, his fortune included six Jamaican estates, which totalled almost 7,000 acres and 457 slaves.

Below are two self-help manuals for healthcare of the enslaved written by Scottish medics. They offer as much advice on efficient exploitation as they do humanitarian care. These pamphlets were published in Britain and were

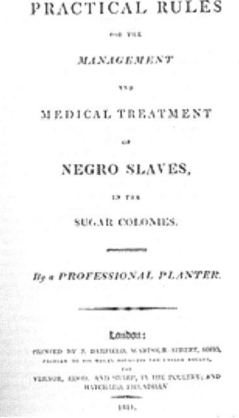

Practical rules for the management and medical treatment of negro slaves

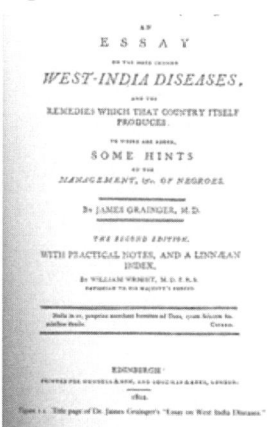

An essay on West India diseases (J. Grainger)

often the subject of debate in medical societies. In Aberdeen and Edinburgh several societies published critiques of the works by physicians who had sojourned in the West Indies.

In 1759 Grainger settled on the West Indian island of St. Kitts, where he married an heiress whom he had met on the voyage out. Not having the funds to set up as a planter himself, he was appointed manager of the family's estates and also continued his medical practice. The practice of medicine alongside other occupations allied to the slave economy was common e.g. plantation, manager, slave ownership and trading.

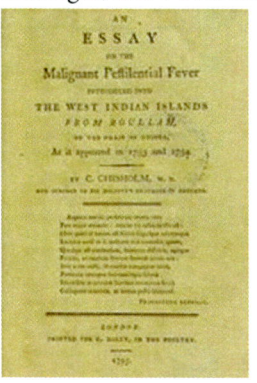

An essay on Malignant Pestilential fever. (Chisolm)

Dr Colin Chisholm of Inverness graduated from Aberdeen University in 1793 and was a medical practitioner in Grenada, landowner in Demerara and the author of an essay on yellow fever. He was one of the first to argue that it was a contagious disease, introduced to the Caribbean through the transportation of slaves from Africa. Later in life he lived in Bristol and sponsored Bristol students who attended the University of Aberdeen.

Examples of Scottish Doctors in the West Indies.

Dr Jonathan Troup (Dominica)

Was born in 1764 in Aberdeen and graduated with an MA from Marischal College Aberdeen in 1786. Following medical studies in Glasgow and Aberdeen, he visited London. In 1790 he was recruited as an assistant by Dr Clarke on the recommendation of Dr Morrison of Aberdeen.

Dr James Clark of Aberdeen owned Clark Hall Estate in Dominica, a sugar plantation, home, at its peak, to 250 slaves. He published a Treatise on the Yellow Fever based on his own observations. The study hypothesised about the reasons for the outbreak and was one of the first studies to hint at the role of mosquitoes in the spread of disease. He also discussed symptoms of the disease and possible means of prevention. The study also branches into commentary on other diseases such as typhus, dysentery, cholera and tetanus. Dr Troup was the assistant of Drs Clark and Finlan whose practice covered two thirds of Dominica's population (1500 European, 14,500 enslaved), the rest were covered by eleven doctors.

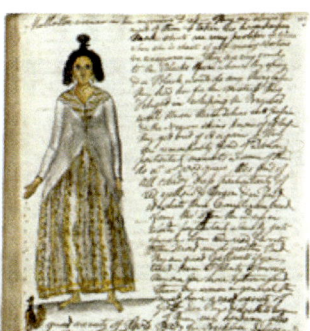

Jonathan Troup Journal, illustrated description of mullato culture.

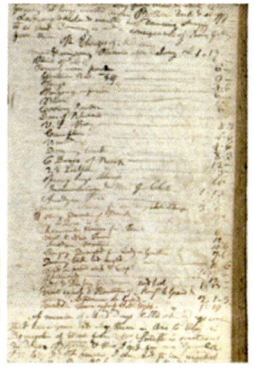

A list of Troup's fees for procedures and medication, Dominica Journal p.94

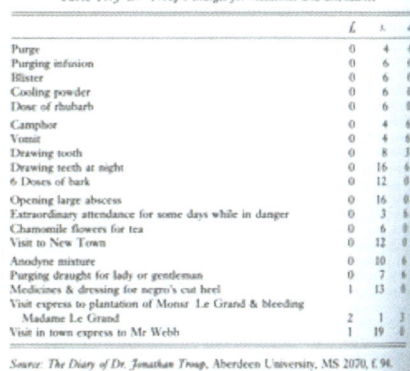

Troup's professional fees

Table 11.3 Dr Troup's charges for medicines and attendance			
	£	s.	d
Purge	0	4	4
Purging infusion	0	6	0
Blister	0	6	0
Cooling powder	0	6	0
Dose of rhubarb	0	6	0
Camphor	0	4	6
Vomit	0	4	6
Drawing tooth	0	8	3
Drawing teeth at night	0	16	6
6 Doses of bark	0	12	0
Opening large abscess	0	16	0
Extraordinary attendance for some days while in danger	0	3	6
Chamomile flowers for tea	0	6	0
Visit to New Town	0	12	0
Anodyne mixture	0	10	6
Purging draught for lady or gentleman	0	7	6
Medicines & dressing for negro's cut heel	1	13	0
Visit express to plantation of Monsr Le Grand & bleeding Madame Le Grand	2	1	3
Visit in town express to Mr Webb	1	19	0

Source: The Diary of Dr. Jonathan Troup, Aberdeen University, MS 2070, f. 94.

In his journal Troup gives insights into the interactions between the enslaved and free populations including those of mixed race(mullato). He includes direct observations such as *"Saw Dr Clark's Negro with a chain and collar of iron round his neck. Though he is strong, the weight made him bleed at nose and mouth. Dr Clark has about 50 Negroes employed – he makes great profits by them."*

The list of Troup's professional fees, shown above, reflects the common treatments of the time; it is compatible with published works of his contemporaries.

Jonathan Troup's Dominican journal supports the views of his contemporaries in several areas. He identified a white ruling society that was close knit, promiscuous, abusive, and overindulgent but also included those who were well read and scientifically curious. He recorded the inter-racial sexual relations ranging from consensual relationships with free mullato mistresses to the abuse of slaves as observed by others. The diseases he encountered and their treatment mirrored that of the pre-scientific medical practice of the late Enlightenment. His drive to obtain a scientific reputation rapidly rather than gradually, as did other doctor naturalists, is evident. The illustrations of the island's flora and fauna are specific to Troup's journals.

Troup's writings and experiences differ from those of most of his contemporaries in several ways. He recorded anthropological details of the enslaved and free people of colour, his observations often supported with illustrations. In particular his recording of an instance of literacy and evidence of voluntary individual Christian witness among the enslaved is unusual. Troup's Dominican journal provides the narrative of a failed West Indian sojourn, giving an alternative insight into the support network so often lauded in Scottish diaspora.

Dr William Wright 1735 – 1819.

Wright's story is not untypical. In 1756, after a surgical apprenticeship, Wright attended medical lectures at Edinburgh University, but did not obtain a degree. In 1757, he sailed to Greenland as a ship's surgeon on a whaler. In 1758, Wright presented himself for examination at the Surgeons' Hall in Edinburgh and was subsequently appointed surgeon's mate on a Royal Navy warship. He returned to Britain in 1763, receiving an MD in absentia from St Andrews University.

Wright left for Jamaica in 1764, hoping to establish a practice there, but there were already too many doctors. He became an assistant on a sugar plantation, where he invested his savings in slave trading. An old friend offered him a partnership in a medical practice at Hampden estate in Jamaica. This practice was responsible for the medical care of 1200 slaves and the local free population. Wright began his study of botany and became a collector of Jamaican plants. In 1774 he was appointed Surgeon-General of Jamaica. in 1777 he left Jamaica for London where he furthered his knowledge of obstetrics, botany and medicine. Wright returned briefly to Edinburgh, attending lectures at Edinburgh University, before embarking again on his travels in 1779. Wright was known as a botanist, collector and naturalist. After medical service with a Jamaican regiment, during war with Spain, he worked in Jamaica from 1782 to 1785. In1785 he returned to Edinburgh, having secured the sale of his property in Jamaica. He occupied himself in Edinburgh's scientific societies and culture. Wright was politically conservative and opposed the abolition of the slave trade.

Conclusion

Scots doctors were involved in the slave trade and the plantation economy. The latter is often forgotten but perhaps represents a longer deep-seated involvement in slavery.

Most Scots were sojourners rather than permanent colonists; their aim was to make sufficient money to gain a comfortable life and position back in Britain. Recruitment depended on professional and kinship networks. Medicine offered a method of economic and social advancement in the plantation society. Many doctors, using their education, multi-tasked, acting as agents for absentee plantation owners or were engaged in slave and plantation owning themselves. Healthcare for the enslaved was mainly motivated by improved commercial exploitation of the slave-based system.

Some colonial doctors used their leisure time not only for medical research but the study of botanical, geographic and ethnological studies. Such activity and resulting publications were typical of the polymaths of the Enlightenment. For those interested in the subject of medical practice in the era of slavery I would recommend the work of Richard Sheridan *"Doctors and Slaves: A Medical and Demographic History of Slavery in the British West Indies, 1680-1834."* And *"Scotland, the Caribbean and the Atlantic World, 1750-1820"* by Douglas Hamilton

Bibliography

- T.M. Devine (ed), Recovering Scotland's Slavery Past, The Caribbean Connection. (Edinburgh 2015)
- D. Hamilton, Scotland, the Caribbean and the Atlantic World, 1750-1820. (Manchester, 2005).
- R. Sheridan, Doctors and Slaves: A Medical and Demographic History of Slavery in the British West Indies, 1680-1834. (Cambridge, 1985).
- S. Schwarz, Slave Captain: The Career of James Irving in the Liverpool Slave. (Wrexham 2008).
- Papers of Jonathan Troup physician of Aberdeen, Scotland and Dominica, West Indies. Aberdeen Special Collections (Reference GB 231 MS 2070). Also available as digitalised images at https://www.abdn.ac.uk/special-collections/.

VESALIUS: A BIOGRAPHY
1514-1564.
Father of Human Anatomy and Surgical pioneer.

Walford Gillison
Presented to the Bristol medico-Historical Society Monday 14 October 2019

Our hero was born into a well to do family based mainly in or around Brussels in what was called Flanders but he described himself as a citizen from the "Low Countries".

Andreas Vesalius.

His actual family name was "Wijtink" but he and the generations before him were known as "Van Wesel". He was christened Andries van Wesel on New Year's Eve in 1514. It turned out to be convenient in his later life when he found his house and grounds were situated near a common field where the City of Brussels public gallows for criminals was situated!

When he was born it was also a time of alternative religious movements, a time of economic and flood disasters which made life even worse after a series of bad harvests for agriculture. It was also a time where there were repeated Bubonic plagues and the dreaded *"English disease"* or the *"Sweating sickness"* (syphilis).

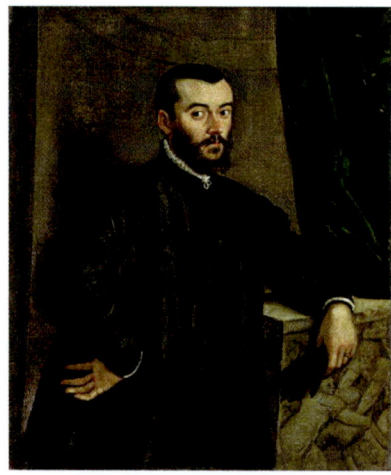

Portrait of Vesalius by Jan Stephen Kalkar.
www.bing.com.images

Our hero, Andries van Wesel Junior, later known all over Europe by his Latinised name as Vesalius was born on New Year's Eve in 1514 into a well-to-do and highly intelligent medical family, four generations of whom had been exposed to the ancient but highly respected Persian medical giants of Rhazes (865-925) and Avicenna (980-1037).

1. *Peter Wesel.* (Great-great Grandfather) This famous forebear was a physician at the University of Padua and personal physician to Emperor Frederick III 1415-1493. Peter Wesel was a renowned expert on the teachings of Avicenna.
2. *Johan van Wesel.* (Great Grandfather) Eminent physician of Brabant and pioneer founder of the School of Medicine of Leuven.
3. *Evaert van Wesel* (Grandfather). Physician and expert on the book "Liber Almansorem" by Rhazes. He also was an expert on the first four parts of the Aphorisms of Hippocrates.
4. *Andries van Wesel. Snr.* (Father). He was Court pharmacist to the current Holy Roman Emperor Charles V.
5. Finally, our hero, *Andries van Wesel Jnr.*

Our hero lived in Europe at the time of four powerful potentates, emperors or dictators. All were about the same age and their ambitions resulted in many deaths and destructions on so many European battlefields. The four men were:

1. Charles Vth. Holy Roman Emperor (1500- 1558).
2. François I of France (1494–1557).
3. Henry VIII of England (1491-1547).
4. Süleyman The Magnificent (1494–1566).

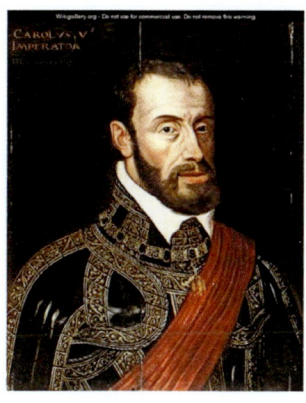

Hapsburg Emperor Charles V
https://www.bing.com/images

Our hero's father was Chief pharmacist at the court of the Holy Roman Emperor Charles V based frequently either in Brussels, Vienna or Rome.

At the age of 16 Vesalius attended the University of Louvain where he was taught subjects including Rhetoric, Grammar and Dialectics.

When older he was taught Greek and Latin so that he could study more original texts from the pioneers from the past. He learned Hebrew as well so as to study the works of a famous Jewish historian who wrote about the great Persian physicians, such as Rhazes and Avicenna. A knowledge of Greek was required for the study of Hippocrates.

In 1533 at the age of 18 he was starting his Medical studies, when at this stage the Emperor Charles advised him to go to the Sorbonne in Paris. He was placed under Jean Fernel for Medicine and Jean Tagault for Surgery, but took extra lessons in a private college under Jacques Dubois (aka Sylvius) who taught straight from the teachings of Galen which had been recently translated from the original Greek into Latin.

Like a surgical dresser or clinical clerk, he was appointed to study under Johann Guinther who incidentally translated some of Galen's anatomical works in 1521. Thus, the fashion among academics was that Galen's works were not "old hat", but "hot news". Soon after his arrival in Paris, Vesalius became dissatisfied with the University tradition of the chaired professor supervising untrained Barber Surgeons who actually did the dirty work conducting the dissection of corpses but mostly animals.

Hence his disparaging comment of Gunther: *"I would not mind as many cuts inflicted upon me as I have seen him make on a man or brute, except at the banqueting table!"* Thanks to his relatively affluent background, Vesalius and some friends resorted to learn human anatomy the hard but costly way.

To do what he wanted he had to:
1. Find money for the hangman and his two assistants.
2. Pay a boatman to cross the Seine from the Gallows field to the Hôpital Dieu.
3. Pay the boatman again to remove the head to avoid identification by relatives.
4. Conduct a clandestine dissection of the corpse in the empty Anatomy theatre at night.
5. Purchase two candles from a local tavern for the corpse's burial service.
6. Pay a priest to conduct the burial service.
7. Finally, clean out the theatre before the Professors arrived in the morning.

This was definitely a winter or low temperature occupation. His habit for studying osteology in summer was by digging out the bones of criminals hanged at Montfaucon then outside Paris. After all, corpses in summer were unbearably smelly without preserving solutions. After consulting his teachers while still a medical student, he got permission to replace the Barber surgeons at the dissecting table so he could learn anatomy with his hands as well as his eyes.

It was in this way Vesalius proved he had the money, the energy and the *"fire in his belly"* to become the worldwide pioneer. Like Leonardo a few years before him, he argued; according to the Catholic Church, convicted criminals were never going to heaven, so they could serve humanity with their bodies after their death.

Meanwhile storm clouds had gathered over Europe because of the death of the Duke of Milan, a shrewd operator who had kept the peace between Charles V and Francis I of France for some time. The control of Milan was an important prize. Therefore, Milan was a prize well worth capture by both powerful potentates and so Charles and Francis were at war again.

As war had been declared by the Holy Roman Empire against France in 1536, Vesalius had to leave Paris in a hurry. And so he returned to the University of Leuven to plan his medical career. While at home he argued against various venesectionists who disputed the merits of whether physicians should take blood from the left arm or from the right arm!

He attended the Countess of Egmond's niece just before she died of respiratory failure due to the wearing of the very tight fashionable chest garment called the Basquine. The garment proved far too tight to allow adequate breathing.

Just before he left home, he somehow obtained a freshly-hanged criminal

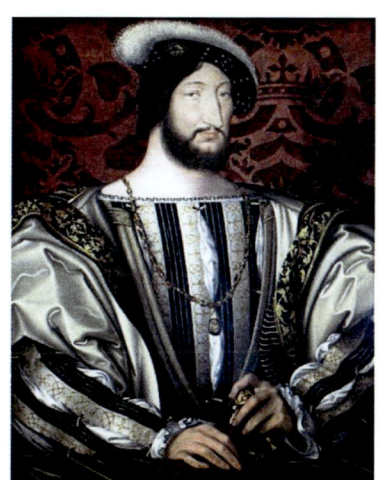

Francis I of France

from the gallows near his home and prepared a fine preparation of the skeleton and presented it to his University Medical faculty.

Vesalius felt he had to proceed to Italy to advance his career. First, he travelled to Venice where he not only met the famous painter Titian but fortuitously met Titian's Flemish student Stephen van Calcar, who was going to help him in a very short time when he reached Padua. While still in Venice Vesalius was impressed by Ignatius of Loyola, the founder of the Jesuit community.

His first moves when he reached the famous University of Padua, was a sequence of assessments and examinations. He sat the University examinations in Padua from December 3rd to 5th in 1537. Found to be outstanding, he was rapidly appointed on December 6th to the post of Prelector in the vacant second Chair of Anatomy and Surgery and given the responsibility of no less than up to 18,000 students.

In the following year in 1538 he started his publications such as *"The Tabulae Anatomicae"* for students which were mainly pictorial, but his real "Magnum Opus" that was going to drastically shake the academic world was the book called *"De humani corporis fabrica libri septem"* ("On the fabric of the human body in seven books"). This was published in 1543. It was a major advance in the history of anatomy over the long-dominant work of Galen, and this book caused tremendous opposition particularly from his old mentor Sylvius in Paris.

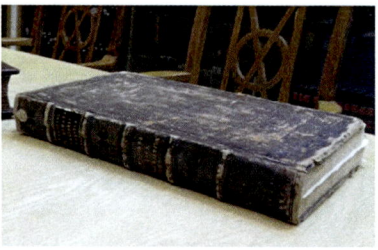

"De humani corporis fabrica libri septem"
"On the fabric of the human body in seven books"
Courtesy RSM library with thanks

There were and thankfully still are, seven sections in his magnum opus *Fabrica*:

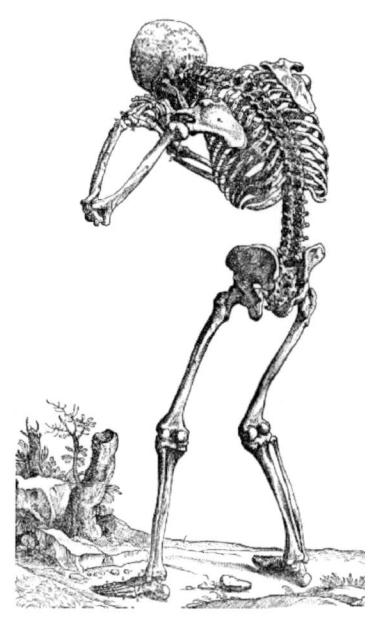

Anterior muscles.

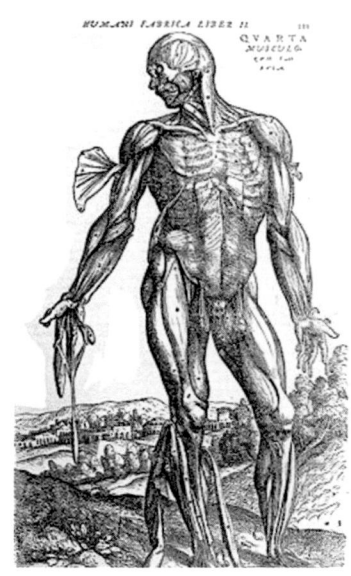

Volume I.   Skeleton.
Volume II.   Muscular system.
Volume III. Veins and arteries.
Volume IV.   Nervous system.
Volume V.   Alimentary tract.
Volume VI. Heart and lungs in particular.
Volume VII. Brain and sensory organs.

His choice of artist in his friend Stephen Van Calcar was fortunate, likewise the choice of publisher who was a Swiss printer called Johannes Herbst (Oporinus), his company performed the woodcuts still beautiful to behold today.

Here are some of the many illustrations, in the book alongside which, printed in a beautiful font, were his descriptions in Latin. For example: *Regarding the human skeleton:* He insisted the students could identify all the bones when blindfolded, they had to distinguish whether the bone was male or female and while still blindfolded, declare which limb bone was from the left side and which from the right!

Here is a wonderful image of the anterior musculature of the human body.

Here below:
 The EXPOSED HUMAN BRAIN

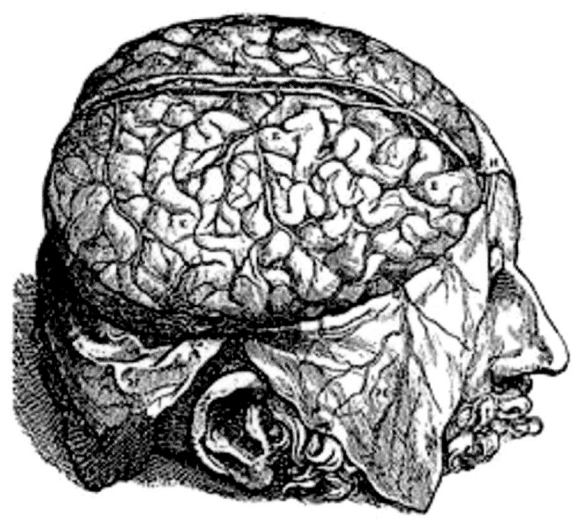

The ABDOMINAL VISCERA including the Appendix

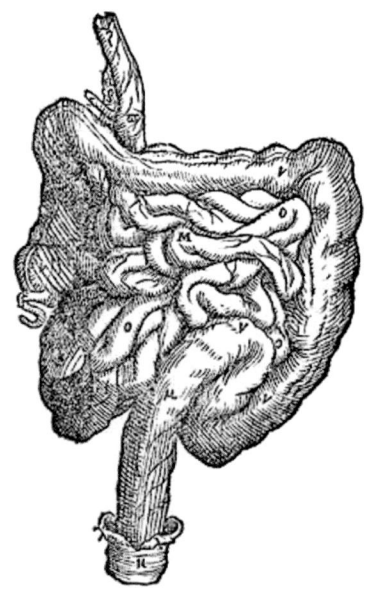

Of special interest regarding this image of the abdomen, this drawing is the second time in history the human **vermiform appendix** has ever been drawn. The first was by Leonardo probably around 1515 shortly before his demise in 1519. Leonardo's famous anatomical drawings had been lost for several centuries until the twentieth century. Therefore, the very existence of the human appendix was not universally known until the drawings presented by Vesalius.

While Galen (130 – 200 AD) had performed many dissections on animals such as the ape which has no appendix, Galen might be forgiven because he was forbidden by his Roman conquerors to dissect or touch human corpses except on the battle field or the stadium.

Vesalius soon published a shorter and cheaper version of *"Fabrica"* for students called *"Epitome"*. His main trouble was the success of the Anatomy triumph was such that plagiarised versions appeared over Europe for financial benefit of the intellectual thieves. The second edition of *Fabrica* was in 1555 maintaining the same high quality of the original.

At this stage our hero was honoured to be invited to take the post of chief physician to the Emperor now engaged in several wars, mostly against Francis I. Added to the Emperor's troubles, because of his strict Catholic faith, Charles V found himself in conflict with the increasing number of German Protestant groups, mainly the Schmalkaldic league, a military alliance of Lutheran princes within the Holy Roman Empire. Although originally started for religious motives soon after the Reformation, this league intended to replace the Holy Roman Empire as chief focus of political allegiance as well.

Vesalius was not perfect and he did make some mistakes:

- He invented a "Retractor Bulbi" muscle in man but this muscle is only present in whales and some other animals.
- Like Galen he believed that blood was made in the Liver. This is understandable after exploring many soldiers for military trauma he would have seen in military service. A ruptured liver bleeds very fast, very profusely and often fatally.
- He described three layers lining human veins.

- He alleged most normal sacral bones had six and not five segments.
- He described the uterus perfectly but omitted the oviducts. These were later named by Gabriele Falloppio who had succeeded him at Padua.

The things which he got absolutely right included:

- He totally debunked the arguments for left and right sided venesections.
- Proved the dangers of Basquine garments in young women as described earlier.
- He demonstrated Galen's errors on so many things, but lacked tact in his writings. For example, he showed the valves of the heart were impermeable in contradiction to Galen.
- He described the anatomy of the human hymen, a structure previously unmentionable in front of the clergy.
- At court in Brussels, he performed open drainage of osteomyelitis of the tibia of the Emperor's Chamberlain with excellent healing. (Centuries before antibiotics).
- He recommended if it were possible, all chronic empyemas around the lung should be drained.
- He was quoted as having said: *"Aristotle and many others say men have more teeth than women: it is no harder for anyone to test this than it is for me to say it is false, since no one is prevented from counting teeth"*.

At this time Sylvius in Paris wrote furiously against Vesalius his former pupil, because Vesalius had suggested much of Galen's work on human anatomy was incorrect. Sylvius excused Galen's errors by suggesting human anatomy had changed over the 1400 years since the great man's death!

Soon after the publication of *"Fabrica"* he joined the Emperor to be chief medical officer on several military campaigns. This offer was so different from teaching anatomy and dissecting the human body, one might suspect his patron's offer was one he dare not refuse.

This experience of active wartime service to the following conflicts must have been tremendous, they included:

1. 1543. Battle of Mainz.
2. 1544. Siege of St Dizier
3. 1544. Battle and Treaty of Crĕpy.
4. 1546-1548. Wars by Charles V against the German Protestants.
5. 1552. Siege of Metz.

His main duties were resuscitation, splinting or amputating broken limbs and if possible, saving lives. Most of the patients mentioned seemed to have had a celebrity status. More frequently his duties in battle were dealing with those that were slain. The deceased had to be eviscerated, their bodies embalmed and then sent home to the families.

In 1544, after the siege of St Dizier he returned to Brussels, sorted his father's legacy after sudden death and got married to Anna Van Hammer. The next year his daughter Anna was born.

In 1556 the Holy Roman Emperor Charles V abdicated following a sequence of military failures, gout, malaria and depression. Therefore, Vesalius was transferred to Charles' son Philip, who detested the Low Countries and Germany, preferring to spend more time in Spain, for example it was he who had sent out explorers like Cortez to the New World.

Vesalius soon learned he was heartily detested by the jealous Spanish physicians in Court in Madrid. Apart from Prince Don Carlos he was only allowed to treat non-Spanish patients. There he met and enjoyed the company of Ambroise Paré who had supported the opposing French troops in previous wars.

In 1559 Philip II married Elizabeth of France and thus ended the war between the Hapsburgs Empire and Kingdom of France. Vesalius was miserable in Spain; he was frustrated he could only treat foreigners in Spain. However, he successfully performed an emergency trephine or craniotomy for post-traumatic osteomyelitis of the forehead of the skull in Prince Don Carlos, son of Phillip II. Despite that timely intervention, the spiteful Spanish court claimed the cure was thanks only to the prayers of the priests that were attending.

After a few uneventful years in Spain in 1564 there came a report that Vesalius was in danger of being executed for a serious crime. There were two very different stories for his being in such danger.

1. He was accused by the Spanish court of conducting a dissection on a human body in which the heart was still beating. It is hard to believe the most knowledgeable anatomist in the civilised world, a man with tremendous military experience of soldiers stricken in battle, would be capable of making such a mistake. It was said too that Philip of Spain intervened and to pacify the critics, requested Vesalius to make penance in the holy Land.
2. Another report suggested he had been very ill in Madrid but thanks to his recovery he vowed to go to Jerusalem to give thanks to the Almighty for his cure.

Whatever the explanation, he decided to leave Spain forever and hopefully return to teaching anatomy preferably in Padua. He took his wife and daughter with him to Venice before despatching them home to Brussels. Meanwhile he took a sea voyage for his pilgrimage to the Holy Land. He did get there successfully because his presence in Jerusalem was witnessed by the Venetian ambassador.

Tragically on the way back to Venice his ship was shipwrecked on the Island of Zante off the west coast of Greece. He was buried in a small chapel on the island but the chapel and his remains were utterly destroyed by two earthquakes in that same year of 1564.

Philip II gave Vesalius' wife Anne a generous pension for the rest of her life.

SUMMARY

Vesalius was born into an intelligent and influential family, no doubt he could have chosen a life of comfort, but he took the hard road to study human anatomy and advance his medical knowledge. To achieve his purpose, he cultivated powerful or useful friends such as Emperor

Charles Vth, Ambroise Paré, Steven Van Calcar & Oporinus. The last two produced the finest book of the Anatomy of the Human body in its time.

He applied his immense energy and enquiring mind to his work and he did not mind getting his hands dirty performing public dissections. All this achievement started from his daily legal and illegal dissections in Paris.

Yes, he could be an *"angry"* man and hated pomposity. (Guinther and Sylvius).

He claimed he was not accustomed to saying anything with certainty after just only one or two observations. He believed *"A knowledge of anatomy is equally important to physicians as it is to surgeons"*.

He is the father of Human Anatomy besides being a fine clinical surgeon.

The Bath War Hospital

FRANCIS DUCK
3 Evelyn Road, Bath BA1 3QF
bathduckf@gmail.com

The Bath War Hospital was one of a large number of hospitals set up throughout Britain during the First World War in order to care for the torrent of military casualties from the trenches of northern France. Early in the war, numerous, sometimes quite small, hospitals were set up, stately homes taking a few casualties or civilian hospitals offering to convert some or all of their wards for military use. These war hospitals supplemented the pre-existing military hospitals, operated by the Royal Army Medical Corps.

By the summer of 1915 it had become clear to the War Office that the current provision of military and war hospitals would soon become inadequate to the task, and means to extend this provision were being explored. Small hospitals in the Bath area, such as the forty-bed facility at Kingswood School, had been established in the early months of the war and two Red Cross hospitals, one in Lansdown Crescent and the second in Bathampton were opened. Lord and Lady Temple had set up a small hospital at Newton Park, using their own funds. The Royal Mineral Water Hospital (Min) in Bath had offered space for military casualties, first closing its female wards to do so, eventually making 120 beds available to long-term casualties suffering from shell-shock and rheumatism. The added capacity recently made available in the 500-bed Beaufort War Hospital in the Asylum in Fishponds would still not be enough in the Bristol area. Many more beds were required.

The War Office had divided the country into Commands. The Southern Command, which stretched from Warwickshire in the north and Berkshire in east and extended down to Cornwall, had its HQ in Salisbury. One Saturday evening in May 1915 a telegram arrived from there on the desk of the Mayor of Bath, Mr Frederick Spear, from Salisbury:

'Additional hospital accommodation urgently required by War Office for wounded from overseas. Buildings or group of buildings capable of taking 500 beds and staff wanted. Large rooms necessary. Equipment and staff should be got locally if possible, but paid for by War Department if necessary. Please wire if you can help.'

The word 'urgently' galvanised action. The following Tuesday, Spiers sent the following reply: *'Royal United Hospital can accommodate 130 at once. Arrangements could be made early next week for about 350 in our Assembly Rooms, or 500 in a group of modern built schools.'*

It turned out that there was not the burning emergency implied by the Salisbury telegram after all. During the next couple of months, negotiations between the city council, representatives of St John's Ambulance, the Red Cross, local hospitals and the Southern Command HQ explored possibilities. Bath was not in a position to offer a single building that could accommodate 500 casualties, which is what the War Office really wanted. Prior Park, already occupied by the army, was considered and rejected. The potential accommodation at the Assembly Rooms was insufficient in size. The War Office then offered to provide new buildings, provided that the committee could identify an appropriate site. A suitable location was found at Summerhill Park, on the northern slopes above Bath. It was chosen by the Bath Committee in part as being conveniently close to the homes of local doctors on Sion Hill and to the market gardens on Primrose Hill. There was a public announcement in mid July. Then the War Office surveyor visited Bath and vetoed the site because of its slope.

The Combe Park site

The Committee had no plan B, and needed one quickly. Within two weeks a replacement site had been identified. The new *'Bath Soldiers' Hospital'* would be built on level open land adjoining Combe Park near Weston village on the western outskirts of the city. (Figure 1). The land was owned by Albert Browning JP, a retired teacher, who by this time was the chairman of the Bath Gas Company. It had been previously part of the Weston Manor lands, the eighteenth century home of the pioneer Bath physician, Dr William Oliver. After Browning had purchased the land he moved in to The Homestead, a large residence on Combe Park, and took over the attached Portway School. He then developed the land, building the large semi-detached houses on both

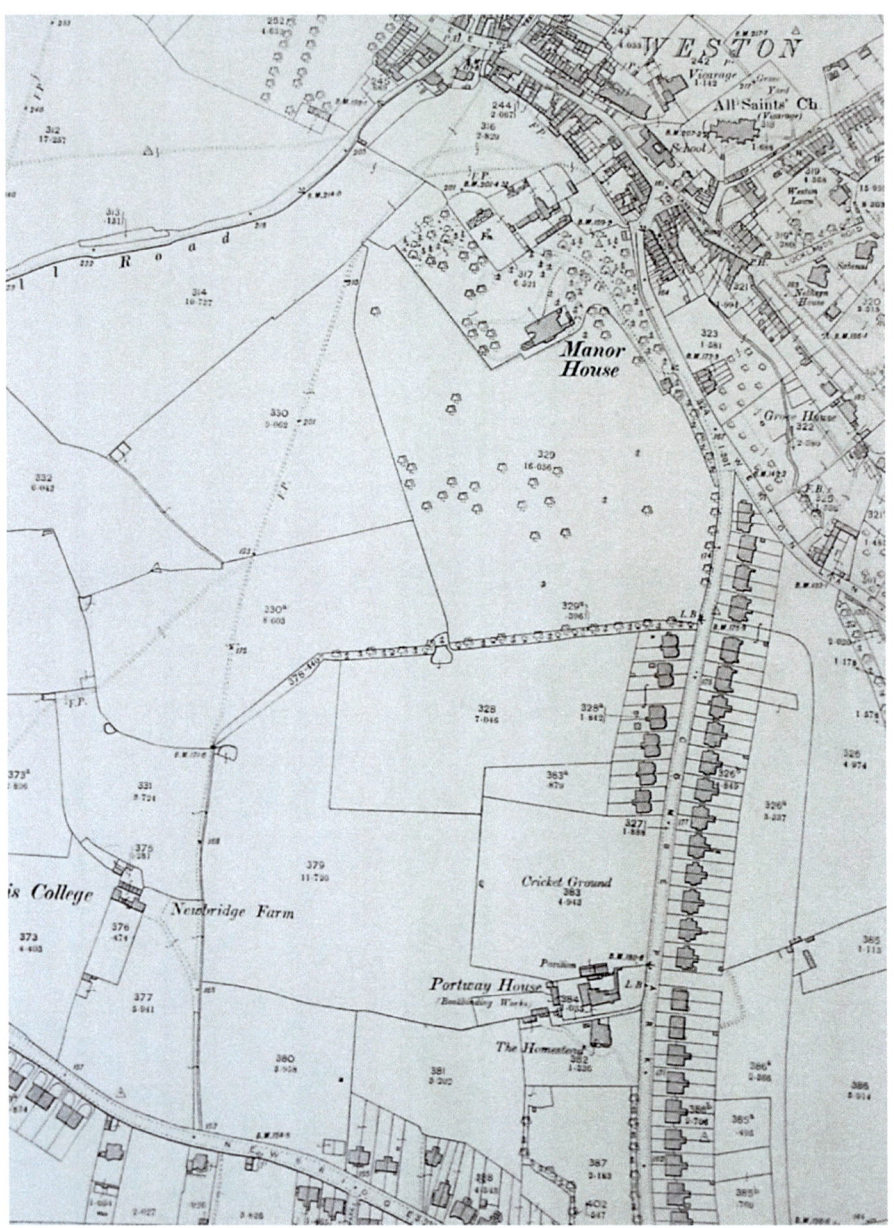

Figure 1. Map of the site of the Bath War Hospital in 1902, showing Combe Park, the Lansdown Cricket Ground, the Portway Bookbinding works and The Homestead.

sides of Combe Park that still remain. The rest of the site was opened for grazing and recreation, sometimes hosting a gymkhana or a visit by the All-England Lawn Tennis and Croquet Club. Of particular interest to this story, he leased the land next to the Homestead to the Lansdown Cricket Club, supposedly the oldest cricket club in Somerset, when it needed to relocate to make way for the Midland Railway at Green Park Station.

The Homestead had than been bought from Browning by another notable Bath personality, Alderman Cedric Chivers, who had developed the adjacent Portway school site to become his internationally-renowned book bindery. It seems very probable that it was Chivers who floated the suggestion that the 80-year-old Browning should sell the rest of his land to the War Office. Browning's only stipulation was that there should be no building on his cherished Lansdown cricket pitch.

The War Office took possession of the 26-acre site on 4th September 1915 and work began in marking out. The design of this and similar temporary war hospitals had been carried out by the Scottish architect Harry Bell Measures FRIBA, Director of Barrack Construction at the War Office, and he visited Bath in its early stages of construction. He was previously known for his design of Rowton Houses, hostels for single men.

It was important to sell the idea to Bath's population, some of whom had already challenged the need and the financial cost that this commitment would bring to the city. The Mayor released a press report in August and then convened a public meeting in October, to convince the waverers. Further encouragement came from Sir Alfred Keogh, the Director of the Army Medical Services, who was:

'greatly in favour of Bath as a place for a military hospital. Its nearness to Southampton, its two railways, and the advantage of the mineral springs placed the city in a most favourable position. In addition to this there was no town the size of Bath with a larger body of resident medical men, physicians and surgeons – the greatest need of all – and this had been a great difficulty in a lot of small hospitals in smaller places.'

Indeed there were plenty of medical men. The 1914 Bath directory lists ninety-seven of them of whom thirty had immediately offered their services to the new hospital.

The hospital required a reliable supply of electricity for lighting and to power the x-ray equipment. Cedric Chivers had his own generator in the Portway bookbinding premises adjacent to the planned site, and this was of sufficient capacity to power the new hospital. Overhead wires were erected to an on-site transformer. This arrangement had an unexpected side effect when a Mr WA Skinner, a married man aged thirty, received his conscription papers shortly after the war hospital opened. Chivers successfully appealed on his behalf, pointing out that Skinner was his employee, responsible for the electrical supply for the hospital x-ray set. He was given *'conditional exemption'*.

Funding and support

The hospital came at an estimated cost to the War Office of £20,000. The committee in Bath undertook to equip the nurses' quarters, the operating theatre and the x-ray room. All the medical staff would be recruited locally, but some would require a *'proportionate salary'*. Nursing staff would also be recruited locally, as far as possible. It was estimated that *'28 trained ladies and 80 voluntary aid ladies'* would be needed. The hospital would be provisioned and maintained locally. The running cost would be about six shillings per day per occupied bed, but only half of this sum would be supported by the War Office, the balance to be found by local fundraising.

This arrangement with the War Office committed the citizens of Bath to raising money to support the hospital. The ladies of Bath, under the lead of the previous mayor's wife Mrs Margarita King and her Needlework Guild, were encouraged to *'fling themselves with the greatest possible ardour into the work of raising the funds while the hospital is being erected'*. Contributions from school bazaars, individual donors and associations were consolidated into a general appeal at the open meeting in October 1915 by the treasurer Walter Mallett, whose wife Margaret would become the catering manager for the hospital. By then, the local Red Cross Society had already committed £1000 to equip the nurses' home and the Somerset Red Cross Society had donated a further £100. A target of over £5000 was set. In truth, some in Bath had been doing quite well out of the war. The local industrialist and munitions supplier, Percy Stothert, told the audience that *'though he was now concerned with making that which caused wounds, he could assure them that assisting in the healing of wounds was a far more congenial task to him'*. In answer to the criticism that there were too many empty military beds already, he went on to argue that *'he had seen enormous extravagance in other directions in this war, but the only extravagance pardonable was extravagance in healing the wounded'*.

Opening, April 1916

By the beginning of April the builders, Wilkins and Sons of Bristol, had completed only half the planned accommodation. Nevertheless, on 8th April, contributors were invited to inspect the new hospital before any patients arrived, even though the main entrance road (Figure 2) had still not been completed. Echoes of this entrance, swinging right then left, just north of the cricket ground, remain still as the entrance to the present A&E department of the Royal United Hospital (RUH). Over 1100 people paid one shilling each to visit.

Ten ward blocks, spaced at 40 ft intervals, were already erected, though only five of these were ready to accept patients. The bare land between them was ready to be laid out with gardens. Each ward was

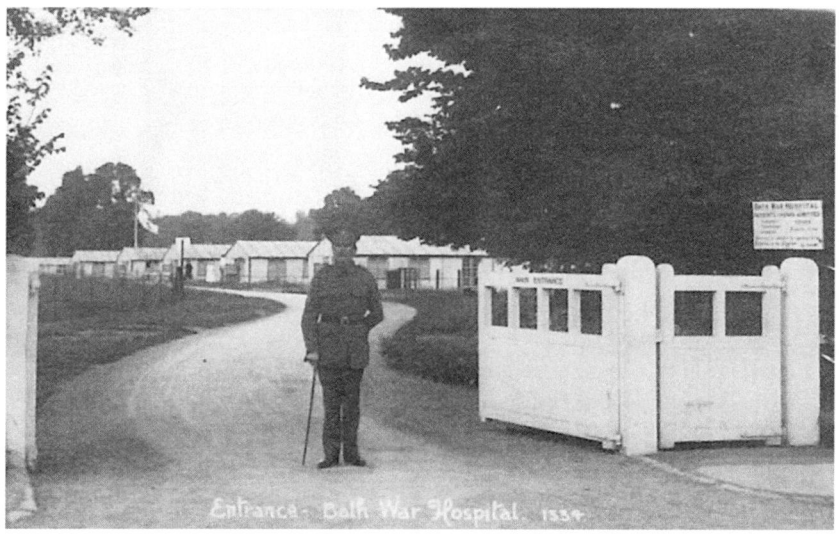

Figure 2. A postcard showing the guarded entrance of the Bath War Hospital, Combe Park

200 ft long and 20 ft wide and was designed to accommodate fifty beds. Constructed of brick and concrete, with asbestos roofs, stained walnut floors and steel framed windows, the interiors were painted *'in a soothing shade of green'*. Electric light bulbs over the beds were alternately open and shaded. The administrative offices, dispensary, clinical laboratory and offices for Commandant and Matron were placed centrally. The operating theatre, x-ray and anaesthetic rooms, and isolation block were at the far end of the 800 ft spine corridor. Stores, kitchen and a dining and recreation room lay to the north. All blocks were connected by telephone.

On-site accommodation for the sixty nurses and assistants was erected towards the south and west of the main wards, in a rectangular arrangement of blocks. It included a separate dining room, kitchen and sick ward. In a remarkable indication of the social background of many nurses, there was also accommodation for sixteen maidservants. Some off-site rooms were also made available for the VADs in Weston Park and Newbridge Hill.

Medical Staff

Twenty-seven Bath physicians and surgeons had finally committed their services to join the honorary medical staff. Particular note will be made of some of these. A complete list is given in Table 1.

Dr Gilbert Bannatyne was appointed to be the Commandant. He had been a physician at the Min from 1894 to 1912. A specialist in the treatment of rheumatoid arthritis, he had published the first x-ray photograph of an affected hand within a year of the discovery of x-rays (1895-96), in his book on the disease. The War Hospital was staffed by civilians, and to ensure appropriate liaison with the military authorities, Bannatyne took a commission as lieutenant-colonel in the RAMC. No other staff members were given military ranks.

Miss Amy Hill, who had been in charge of nursing at the Lansdown Place *'No 2 Red Cross Temporary Hospital'*, was persuaded not to move to St Aldham's House, Frome, which had been taken over as a military hospital, and was appointed to be the matron. She brought military nursing experience, having served in the South African War.

Table 1. Honorary medical staff at the Bath War Hospital when it was opened in April 1916.

Name	Title
Lt-Col Gilbert A Bannatyne MD FRCPE	Commandant
Edward J Cave MD FRCP	
William P Kennedy BA MD BCh BAO Dub	
Thos Wilson-Smith MD MRCS MRCPE	
Charles Begg MB CM Edin	
Norman Lavers MD MRCS LRCP	Psychiatrist
Charles J Whitby MD	
George J Scale MRCS (retired)	Resident medical officer
Alexander L Mackenzie LRCP	
J Maurice Harper MRCS	
Frederick G Thompson MA MD MRCP	
Alfred L Fuller FRCSI MRCS LRCP	
Charles Curd MRCS LSA	
Richard JH Scott FRCSE MRCS	
William H Cooke MD FRCSE MRCS LRCP	
Frederick Lace FRCS LRCP	
James Lindsay MD MRCP	Radiographer
Henry Terry FRCSE MRCS LSA	
Gilbert J King Martyn MD BCh DPH,RCPS	Rehabilitation
Albert E Norburn MD BS MRCS LRCP	
D Leslie Beath MRCS LRCP	Ward doctor
John MH Munro DSc MRCS LRCP	Pathologist
Ray Edridge MRCS LRCP	Anaesthetist
Preston King BA MD MRCS	Radiographer
William H Symons MD MRCS LRCP DPH	Sanitation
Mary EH Morris MD	Medical and surgical registrar
E Whiston	Dispenser

John Munro, the pathologist, was the most academic of the medical staff. His had been a late entry to medicine following a research career in agricultural chemistry. He took responsibility for the laboratory where his bacteriological and biochemical expertise was of considerable value. Many of the patients were suffering from some form of infection, either systemic or local, and Munro's skill in the identification of tetanus, gas gangrene or streptococcal organisms in septic wounds would have been essential.

When the hospital opened, the radiologists were Preston King and James Lindsay. In the press report they were referred to as *'radiographers'*, a general name to describe any who took x-ray pictures. Preston King had arrived in Bath in 1890 as the resident medical officer at the Min. He had introduced radiology to the Royal United Hospital in 1901, and supported the widely-held view that it was radium that caused the therapeutic efficacy of the Bath waters. Apart from his position as a prominent member of the medical community in Bath, Preston King had a significant civic role. He was mayor of Bath at the outbreak of war in 1914, and again during the final year of the war from 1917 to 1918. As noted above, his wife also contributed to the war effort. James Lindsay had been appointed as honorary pathologist at the Min in 1909, where he had introduced radiology in 1911 with his colleague James MacKay. He was amongst the younger doctors, and in August he was called up into the RAMC to take a position in France. Both Preston King and Lindsay would have had to master the techniques for x-ray localisation, widely introduced during the war to assist surgery for the extraction of shrapnel and bullets.

Lindsay was not the only doctor who left to work nearer the front. Another younger man, Ray Edridge, was the anaesthetist at both the War Hospital and at the RUH. There was considerable concern when, in July 1917, he received instructions to join the RAMC in northern France. His departure would leave not only the War Hospital but also the RUH without a lead expert in anaesthetics. Such was the concern that the Chairman of the Board wrote to the Prime Minister, Lloyd George, with a request to intervene. This was, of course, to no avail, and anaesthetics in Bath was left in the less experienced hands of the remaining surgical team. The departure of younger doctors to the front was a real problem for the maintenance of civilian hospital care. The number of honorary consultant doctors at the RUH shrunk from a complement of seventeen at the start of the war to only seven by the middle of 1917. Most of the doctors who served overseas returned safely, but one, the pathologist Dr Almond, was killed in France.

The only woman on the medical staff was Mary Morris, listed as *'medical and surgical registrar'*. Mary Morris was born in Wales and trained in Bristol, one of the very early women to do so. She arrived in Bath in 1908 on a research project at the Min, and set up in practice in Pulteney Street as the first woman doctor in Bath. By 1910 she was London Commandant of the St John's Ambulance Women's VA. In 1912 she had replaced the ageing Medical Officer for Health, William Symons, as Schools Medical Officer. She joined the Bath War Hospital with experience of military casualties, having been one of the physicians at the Newton Park hospital at the beginning of the war.

Another of the Min physicians, Dr Gilbert King Martyn, had been appointed there in 1913 following Preston King's move to the RUH. King Martyn was concerned with the long-term rehabilitation of soldiers in both the Bath War Hospital and the Min and wrote one of the few accounts of the treatment of chronic disabilities in soldiers from the front, published in the Proceedings of the Royal Society of Medicine in January 1917. In his account he describes the treatment of 1390 invalided soldiers using the Bath waters in the Min, of whom 1180 had been discharged *"relieved"* to return to their units or other war work. A few came from the Bath War Hospital. These men suffered from *'the whole gamut of those diseases of "rheumatic" nature produced by damp, cold and injury, fibrositis and perineuritis being the most numerous'*. His involvement with rehabilitation at the War Hospital will be further detailed below.

Casualties arrive

The first convoy of about 100 casualties arrived by a Red Cross train on Easter Monday 24 April 1916. There was no national rail service, so the journey from Southampton was broken at Wimbourne, where the Great Western handed over to the Somerset and Dorset. The arrival at Midland Station was greeted by a reception committee led by the

Mayor of Bath, and cheering crowds. Some twenty-five were stretcher cases, requiring transport by ambulance. The remainder were taken to Combe Park by a fleet of cars. A steady stream of casualties followed, and the hospital beds filled. Thirty-nine Convoys arrived during the first eighteen months. They were received into the hospital by the Men's Detachment, VAD, Somerset No 35, under their Commandant Mr CW Adams.

Little specific detail is known about the medical conditions of the Bath casualties. This is because because all the official records associated with the Bath War Hospital, together with those from all other military and war hospitals, were destroyed after the war. Glimpses remain from other records. One convoy arrived in which all the casualties had been exposed to mustard gas. In another, half the soldiers needed treatment for trench foot. Gwen Malcolm, one of the VADs, wrote of nursing a soldier with gas gangrene infection in his lungs, and of the stench this caused. Another VAD, Kathleen Ainsworth, in a letter to her parents, wrote how the men arrived covered in mud direct from the front, and how impossible they were to clean. King Martyn considered it worthwhile to write to the BMJ in September 1916 to record fifteen patients who had returned from France to Bath with symptoms of malaria. He pointed out that *'the long immunity from malaria enjoyed by this country tends to make us forget the necessity for excluding its presence'*. In due course, Bath would become a local centre for the treatment of tropical diseases in returning soldiers.

Q Block

Without supporting documentation it is not possible to know, for example, how many and what type of operations were carried out, how many arrived with infectious diseases, nor how numerous were those with trench foot or shell shock. For only one department do we have exact numbers, and this was for the physiotherapy department.

Photographs of front-line hospitals commonly emphasise the dead and dying: equivalent photographs in war hospitals back in Britain showed wards full of recovering soldiers. Of the soldiers who made it back to hospitals in Britain, the majority recovered sufficiently to go back to the trenches. The military/medical challenge was two-fold: to return to fitness those who were still able to operate as soldiers in battle, and to rehabilitate the remainder to re-enter civilian life. Dealing with them involved rehabilitation on an industrial scale.

This was not a medical or surgical matter familiar to many civilian doctors, who were more used to treating acute illness. It drew more on techniques used when managing patients with chronic illnesses such as paralysis or rheumatism. So it emerged that the methods used in the middle-class health spas such as Bath were those that were adapted and developed as the main means to rehabilitate the wounded.

A physiotherapy department was not part of the standard design for war hospitals. The idea for a special unit, known as Q-Block, to house a physiotherapy department arose from discussions between Cedric Chivers and his old friend John MacAlister. A Scot who had abandoned his medical training due to ill health, MacAlister was by this time librarian of the Royal Society of Medicine, and secretary of the War Office Surgical Advisory Committee, a service for which he was later knighted. Chivers and MacAlister had become close friends through their common enthusiasm for books, one a bookbinder the other a librarian. They met through the Library Association, and sometimes made family holidays together. With no knowledge of military medicine, Chivers sought MacAlistair's advice on how best he could assist further with the War Hospital in Bath, now that it was operational. MacAlister knew from his London experience that the main function of war hospitals was in the rehabilitation of recovering soldiers, for which a fully equipped department designed to meet this need was an essential component. Chivers had the wealth and motivation to act on this advice.

Q-Block was opened on 19 Nov 1916, at a total cost to Chivers of £1200. Over 100 new patients were treated each month during the next two years. The Bath department was equipped to offer therapy in four categories, as a supplement to manual massage. These were mechano-therapy, electro-therapy, heat and light therapy and hydrotherapy. Evidence for the work of the department arises from three sources, King Martyn's paper in Proc. Roy. Soc. Med. previously mentioned, articles in the Bath Chronicle, and most particularly from a

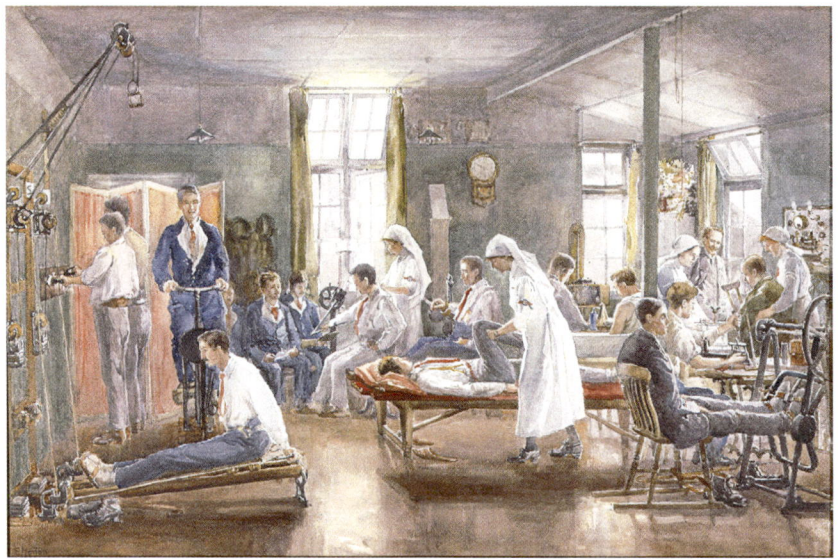

Figure 3. Ettie Horton's watercolour of the interior of Q-Block, c. 1919. Wellcome Library, London.

watercolour painted just after the war by the Ettie Horton, a Bath-based artist otherwise known for her portrayals of landscapes and urban scenes. (Figure 3), This painting is now held by the Wellcome Library in London. Dr King Martyn, the physician placed in charge of the unit, may be seen on the right. Marjorie Cook, the senior masseuse, is placed centrally.

Mechano-therapy

The pieces of equipment shown in Ettie Horton's picture were made by Albert Jones, the engineer of the Corporation Baths, and Ben Smith of Widcombe. The exercise machines were described by King Martyn as comprising a *'carefully planned Zander Institute'*, referring to a form of mechanical exercise pioneered in Sweden at the end of the nineteenth century. Drawings of the workshop designs for some of this equipment, including in some cases the actual dimensions, are attached to the back of the painting. One example, a device for exercising weak thumb and fingers, is shown in figure 4. Others drawings show equipment for rotation of the wrist and the ankle, for flexion and extension of the ankle, fingers, elbow, or knee and for stretching contracted hamstrings. The exercise bicycle was fitted with a simple ergometer.

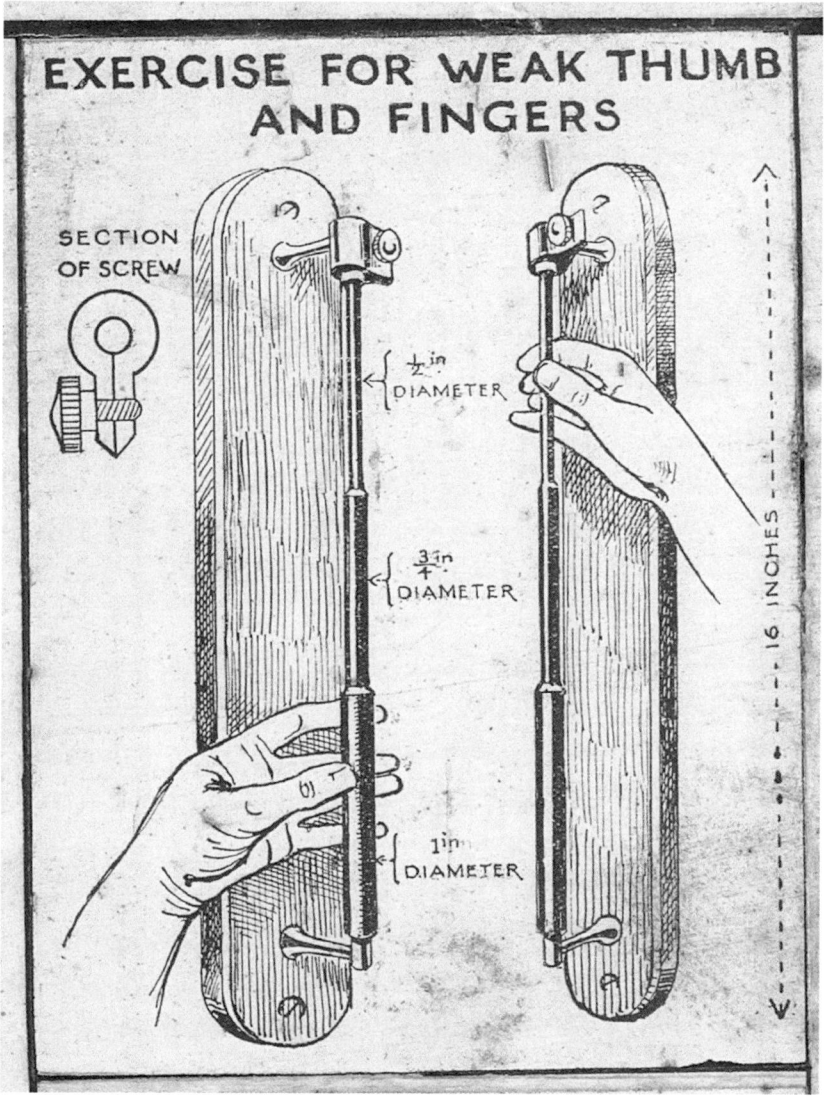

Figure 4.
Design for strengthening exercises for the thumb and fingers.
Mounted on the back of Figure 3. Wellcome Library, London.

Electro-therapy

'*The French War Office considers that the wounds of this great War call for electrical treatment on a wholesale scale*', the words of Dr Ettie Sayer, reporting in 1915 to the Electro-Therapeutical section of the RSM after her recent visit to France. Electrotherapy was also well established in Britain, where the Incorporated Society of Trained Masseuses offered an examination in the Theory and Practice of Medical Electricity, which qualified the successful candidate to '*apply such treatment under the direction of a Registered Medical Practitioner*'. The RAMC was less obviously enthusiastic than the French, although pockets of effective electrotherapy for wounded soldiers, such as that in Q-Block, were established in several war hospitals in Britain.

The British reticence had some justification. Some uses of medical electricity that had been used in civilian practice before the war were of doubtful therapeutic value. The evidence about the Bath War Hospital suggests that Majorie Cook and Dr King Martyn selected those uses of electrotherapy that had by then been shown to have true potential therapeutic effects.

Possibly the most innovative application is almost hidden at the back centre of the painting. The use is more clearly seen in Figure 5, a newspaper photograph taken in Q-block after the war had ended. In this approach, a mechanical metronome was used to interrupt the voltage about once every second, a voltage that was high enough to cause muscle contraction. The wires were usually connected using arm-baths or leg-baths of saline. For soldiers paralysed from damaged but patent motor nerves, interrupted electrotherapy was used to maintain muscle function until nerve control returned. The induced repetitive muscle contraction helped to stimulate circulation and muscle bulk and strength, especially where motor nerve damage made mechanical exercise against weights or using a static bicycle either difficult or impossible.

The other application, mentioned by King Martyn, but not shown in the painting, was ionic therapy. The purpose was to enhance the transport of ionic therapeutic agents through the skin. A high dc current, 50 to 100 mA, was applied over a large area for periods of up to 30 minutes. Metal electrodes up to 10 cm square were covered

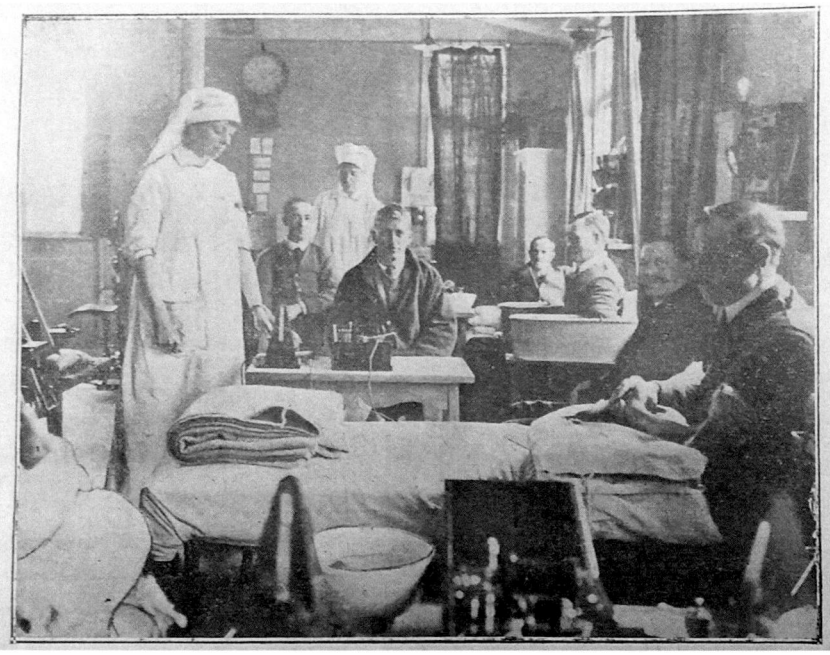

Figure 5. Interrupted electrotherapy in Q-Block, administered by Marjory Cook and Miss Crees. Bath Weekly Chronicle. March 1919.

in several layers of felt, soaked in the appropriate ionic solution and applied to the region to be treated. The drugs most often used were the chlorides of sodium, and lithium and ammonium (for scar softening), sodium zinc sulphate (to treat wounds and ulceration), salycilate (for pain relief), and cocaine hydrochloride (for local analgesia). Ionic medication became less popular after the war, largely because burns from high local currents could occur if the skin was not prepared sufficiently well or the electrodes were applied badly.

Hydrotherapy

The specific physical therapy for which Bath was famed was hydrotherapy. There being no facility for hydrotherapy on the Bath War Hospital site, a few soldiers were occasionally transported to the Min where numerous forms of treatment, used for civilian treatment before the war, were available. One form of hydrotherapy that was available, however, in a room off Q-block, was the whirlpool bath, an early form of Jacuzzi. There were two of these baths, a deep one for legs and a shallower one for arms, purchased from Shanks of Birmingham. Hot water was swirled by means of an electrically-driven turbine in the base of the bath, overlain with a grid for safety. At the same time, bubbles were pumped in through small holes.

Light and radiant heat therapy

The electricity supply made it possible to include two other therapies. On the right of Ettie Horton's painting, beneath the electrical control panel and overseen by King Martyn, she showed an older patient being illuminated with an incandescent bulb. Such therapies were popular, although any benefit accrued from placebo rather than physical effects. More useful were radiant heat baths, in which part of the body, limb or trunk, was enclosed within a metal reflector that was heated electrically to raise the local temperature. Taking advantage of the local workshop, Marjorie Cook designed a radiator for back treatment, which, it was claimed, was effective in cases of lumbago.

By September 1918, shortly before the end of the war, a total of 49,305 treatments from all these techniques were recorded as being applied in Q-Block.

A Growing Hospital

The Bath War Hospital received casualties from the front for two-and-a-half years. Five hundred beds were soon insufficient and the first tents were erected to accommodate 144 more beds in September 1916. Schools in Twerton were considered to take further casualties, but it was decided not to use them. The following February, probably in preparation for the 1917 summer offensive, the War Office decided to double the capacity, supplying marquees and tents to accommodate not only more casualties, but also the staff to tend to their needs.

Figure 6 shows some of this extra accommodation in tents erected on the land to the west of the cricket ground. This image is from one of the postcards that were sold to soldiers to send to their loved ones, and which remain an important record of the War Hospital. The hospital expanded further until, at its largest, the Combe Park site held as

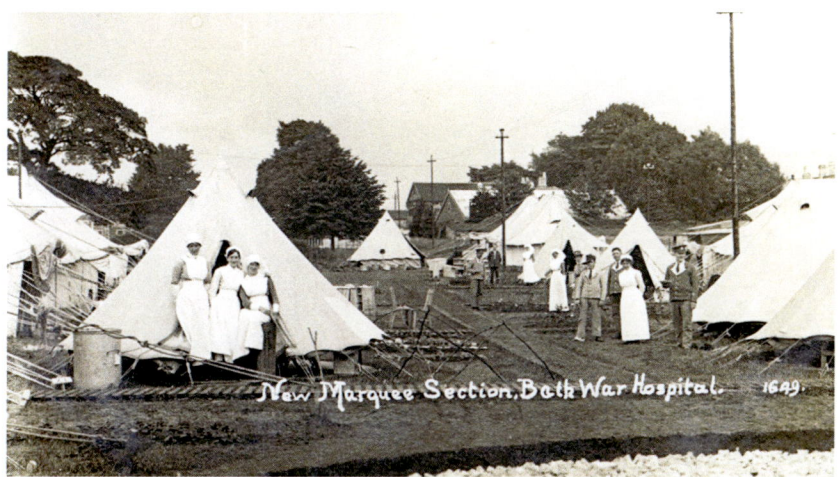

Figure 6. Tented extension to Bath War Hospital, west of the cricket ground showing the electricity cables from the Portway Works. 1917.

many as 1,300 beds. Further accommodation was used in the smaller Bath hospitals when necessary, including a 43-bed ward in the RUH. At its greatest capacity, 1800 casualties were accommodated in Bath, administered from the War Hospital, and accounting for over 3% of the national total. The logistics of managing a temporary hospital of this size stretched the staff to the limit. The number of qualified nurses was increased to fifty. Periodic instructions arrived from HQ to clear beds, anticipating a new influx from the next offensive in France. In August 1917, 700 beds were cleared, about half the hospital capacity, in preparation for the wounded from Third Battle of Ypres. All soldiers who could were moved on to convalescence. They were not transferred to hospitals local to Bath however. In an arrangement that only the army could have invented, Bath War Hospital had been assigned to the 4th General Hospital in the Southern Command. The headquarters was in Plymouth, which was where convalescing soldiers were shipped when space for new casualties was required.

Some soldiers stayed for weeks, and possibly months, especially during the quiet times. The citizens of Bath became familiar with the blue uniforms of soldiers in treatment, as they came in to town for a break or for entertainment.

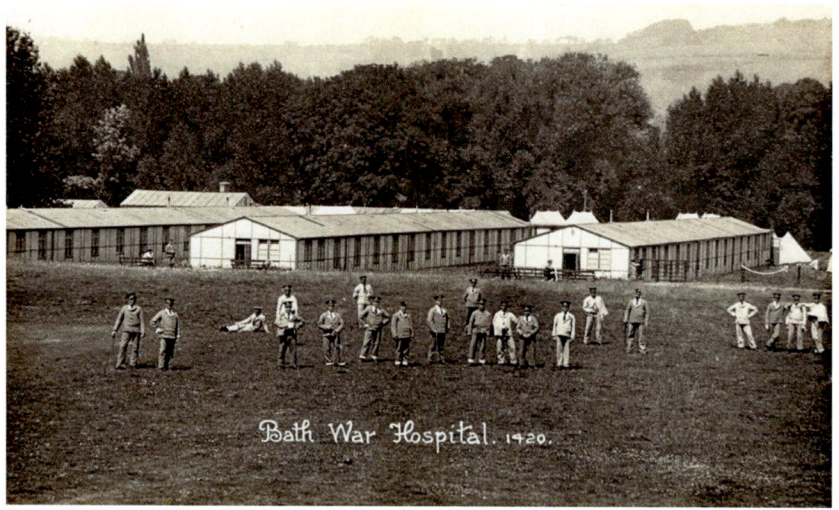

Figure 7. The ward blocks looking north over the cricket ground.

These men found activities to occupy their minds and bodies. The cricket ground gave space for recreation (Figure 7), where they could play football, skittles, and the popular spiro-pole, encouraged by the physiotherapists because it exercised the arm and shoulder muscles. A hospital magazine, the Bath Bun, was published and sold to raise funds. A few items of needlework still remain, some pieces beautifully stitched by individual soldiers with a rare craftsmanship. A competition for the best garden was organised in the summer of 1917 that was won by Ward 1.

Once they were deemed fit for discharge, each soldier left the hospital, either to return to the front, or to one of the army convalescent hospitals, or to be pensioned off. Remarkably few died in Bath, and those that did were buried locally. The graves of these ninety soldiers lie in Locksbrook Cemetery, just off Combe Park, forty-four in a plot managed by the War Graves Commission. Seven Australians and four Canadians were laid to rest far from home. The bodies of the few American soldiers who died in Bath during the winter of 1917-18 were disinterred and returned to their home country.

The Bath Surgical Requisites Association

The support from the citizens of Bath came in two forms, financial and practical. Fundraising continued throughout the war. It had the unforeseen effect of undermining the charitable donations made to the Royal United Hospital which, with its severely curtailed work-force, continued to struggle to meet the medical needs of Bath citizens. By 1918 Dr Preston King, who had been by then re-elected for his second term as Mayor, recommended that Bath's church-going citizens should dig deeper into their pockets each Sunday to ensure that their own RUH remained solvent.

In parallel with the fundraising, a new organisation was established to provide practical help in dealing with the needs of the War Hospital. This was the Bath Surgical Requisites Association, opened in January 1918 with Margarita King, (Mrs Preston King, the lady Mayoress) as president and Cedric Chivers as vice-president. The offices were set up in Chivers' previous bookshop at 39 Gay Street. The unit was the Bath branch of a national organisation, originally part of the Queen Mary's Needlework Guild, which mobilised local volunteers to

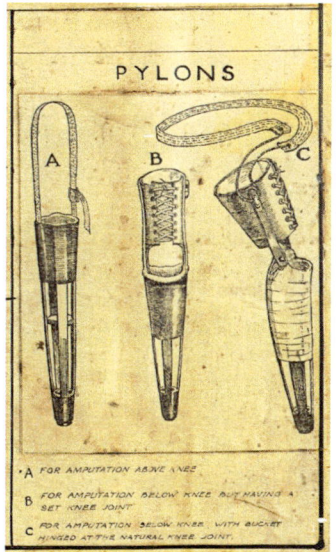

make, initially, bandages and slings, and subsequently made crutches, splints, and other orthopaedic items. In Bath, at least one hundred and seventy local helpers included carpenters who turned peg-legs, known as pylons, for lower limb amputees to wear while they waited to be fitted with full prostheses at Roehampton. (Figure 8) Students at the Somerset Industrial School were set to work turning the ends. The Bath unit was so successful that, by the end of the war, it was one of only six in the country notified by the Joint War Committee to make provisional limbs, the other five being at Alderhay, Liverpool, Ipswich, Kensington and Hove.

Figure 8. Pylons for various levels of amputation.
Mounted on the back of Figure 3. Wellcome Library, London.

Other help came from the local pharmacists, who made thousands of gallons of 'Dakin's Solution', a weak hypochlorite solution that was widely used as an antiseptic in the treatment of deep lacerated flesh wounds. The wounds were continuously irrigated from tanks of the solution mounted above each bed.

Closure

The Bath War Hospital formally closed on 31st December 1919 although, as we shall see, its successors remain on the Combe Park site to this day. Casualties had continued to arrive during the year after the armistice and it was not until 3rd March 1919 that Preston King advised the RUH that he was available to resume his duties as radiologist there. The last of a wartime total of 124 convoys arrived in Bath on 30th June. Bannatyne stepped down as Commandant in July, and Major RM Dickson took over for the last six months. Beneath clear skies in August a sports day was reinstated on the Lansdown Cricket Ground. By the end of the year the temporary tented accommodation had been removed, returning the hospital's nominal capacity to its original five hundred beds.

24,333 cases had been treated since April 1916. The closure was marked by a little gathering in the chapel at which a letter from the War Office was read to the assembled War Hospital Committee, requesting *'that you will be good enough to convey the thanks of the Army Council to the staff of the hospital for the whole-hearted attention and devotion which they have given to the patients who have been under their care'*.

Shortly thereafter the chapel was bought by the Keynsham Rural Deanery for £53 4s and the building was moved to Hampstead Road Brislington.

The question remained: what would happen to the Combe Park hospital site when the War Office no longer needed it? The RUH, which was still housed in its nineteenth-century buildings in Beau Street, was in dire financial straights, with a working loss during 1919 of £5,495 on top of a debt carried over of about £20,000. A transfer to the Combe Park site could release the current building for development, and enable a brand new hospital to be built on the outskirts of the city. Funding would be a problem to complete the move, of course. So, rather than doing it all at once, the first portion of the scheme involved building a

98-bed hospital for paying patients together with a 44-bed maternity home. The land value was estimated to be £6000, but the estimated total cost would be £148,000, a not insignificant sum to raise. It was anticipated that income from these hospitals would begin to stabilise the financial situation. The Hospital Board had been assured by the Department of Health that there was no intention to make hospitals into centrally-funded State hospitals, and that voluntary subscriptions remained the best means of funding, in the government's opinion. That being so, the citizens of Bath were once more to be approached for charitable support, although the outstanding debt was in due course partly paid off from the National Relief Fund. As will be reported next, this plan had to be postponed and it would be another five years before any progress was made. Meanwhile, the government had its own plans for the Combe Park site.

The Pensions Hospital

Closure of the Bath War Hospital, and numerous similar hospitals around the country, did not mean that there were no more war casualties who needed medical care: Far from it. The medical legacy was huge. In April 1920 it was estimated that there were still 24,145 active or pensioned soldiers in or awaiting treatment nationally. Disabled and crippled men needed continuing care and rehabilitation into civilian life. Amputees needed prosthetics. Those suffering from shell shock needed mental care. Many soldiers, otherwise undamaged, returned from the trenches with a variety of chronic pulmonary or neuro-muscular conditions. The government was required to care for these men, under the military pensions scheme. At the end of 1919, responsibility for this care transferred from the War Department to the Ministry of Pensions. A site for a Pensions Hospital for the south west was sought.

For a while during the war the Beaufort War Hospital had been a military orthopaedic centre. As the numbers of amputees increased, with their continuing need for orthopaedic care, a larger facility was opened at the Bristol Military Hospital at Southmead. In the eyes of those responsible for planning, this made Southmead a suitable place to house a Pensions Hospital. Unfortunately the Bristol Guardians, who had been happy to re-house their patients from Southmead Workhouse when the army took it on, now needed urgently to recover the building to house their Bristolian 'sick paupers'. The Bath War Hospital site offered an attractive alternative, because there were no prior claims for its use. As a result, when the existing Bath War Hospital buildings were released from the War Office at the end of 1919, they were simply transferred to the Ministry of Pensions, and Bath became the main military surgical and rehabilitation centre for the whole of the South West of England. The site was sufficiently spacious to still allow the Royal United Hospital to lease land on the south of the site for their private hospital and maternity home.

Nurses from the Bath War Hospital were transferred to the Ministry of Pensions Nursing Service. A few physicians, surgeons and masseuses came over from Bristol, some from the RAMC team in Southmead. They were led by the pioneering orthopaedic surgeon Ernest Hey-Groves, who became the surgical director. He brought his senior registrar from Bristol General Hospital, Duncan Wood, and the ENT surgeon Andrew Wright, also from the BGH. The new Commandant was initially Lieut.-Col. Milne-Thompson, followed by Col. Hubert A Bray in 1923. Miss Maud Ellen Tait was appointed as matron with a nursing staff of seventy-five. Anaesthetics, radiology and pathology were provided by visiting Bath doctors. A complete list of medical staff is given in Table 2. None of the war-time Bath doctors remained, and the new visiting civilian doctors were all given military ranks to work alongside their RAMC colleagues from Bristol.

The operating facilities were upgraded to include a second theatre to be reserved for septic cases to minimise the risk of cross-infection. Technically challenging operations including bone grafting and ophthalmic surgery were introduced. A new, larger physiotherapy department was opened to replace Q-Block, funded by the Long Ashton Division of the British Red Cross Society, and presented by its vice-president Mrs George Gibbs CBE of Tyntesfield. At the same time, the Ministry of Pensions sanctioned the Bath Hospital to become a full artificial limb centre, no longer limited to the construction and fitting of provisional 'pylons', extending the reach of the Bath workshops to include the greater technical challenge of prescribing, fitting and repairing prosthetic legs and arms for all levels of amputation. No

	Name	Title
Full-time RAMC	Lieut-Col Alexander Milne-Thompson CMG MB CM	Medical superintendant
	Major William A Holland MRCS LRCP	Medical registrar
	Capt Harry H Butcher MRCS LRCP	Out-patient department
	Capt C Vandrey Cant	Senior medical officer
	Capt Chas H Hart MB ChB	
	Capt John S Levis MC MB BCh	Anaesthetist
	Capt Reginald B Britton MRCS LRCP	
	Capt H Charlton	Neurologist
	Capt JS Gilbert	Surgeon, limb-fitting department
Visiting	Ernest W Hey-Groves MD MRCS LRCP	Surgical director
	Wilfred G Mumford, OBE MB FRCS LRCP	Surgeon
	Forbes Fraser, CBE FRCS MRCS LRCP	Surgeon
	Duncan Wood FRCS	Surgeon
	Ronald G Gordon MD BSc MRCPE	Neurologist
	Rupert Waterhouse MD MRCP	Pathologist
	James F Mackay MD MB BCh	Radiologist
	Andrew J Wright MB BCh	ENT specialist
	Arthur de V Blathwayt MRCS LRCP	Anaesthetist
	AJ Bruce Leckie MD BCh	Anaesthetist
	Ernest W Witham MRCS LRCP	Tropical diseases
	A Beck Cluckie MB ChB	Ophthalmologist

Table 2 Medical staff of the Bath Pensions Hospital when it was opened in 1920. The military ranks awarded to the visiting medical staff have been omitted. Milne-Thompson was replaced by Col. Hubert Bray CB CMG in 1923. William Beaumont, eye specialist and James Payne, ward master, joined later.

longer would servicemen from the south west have to join the queue for fitting at Roehampton.

The obvious initial priority, other than in othopaedics, was for neurasthenic and tropical disease patients, and the initial plan was to use all five hundred beds for these three specialties only. A short-lived hospital of 120 beds was also established at Ashton Gate, but otherwise Bath became the only centre to treat army pensioners in the south west. By the summer of 1920, the medical need had become much clearer. The focus had moved away from mending broken limbs and minds. Only fifty beds were reserved for neurological patients and eighty for orthopaedics, including the beds at Ashton Gate. The remaining beds were categorised as being for *general and surgical* patients. A separate ward was built to house thirty patients with tropical diseases, with Bath also receiving referrals from Wales. This unit was headed by Ernest Witham, appointed by the Ministry of Pensions as the specialist in tropical diseases. A veranda was commissioned for the open-air treatment of patients suffering from TB. Army pensioners suffered from the same spectrum of diseases as the general public.

Nevertheless, there remained a strong focus on the need to give amputees the skills to enable them to re-enter civilian life. In support of this objective, nearly a dozen remedial workshops were opened. These were initially under the direction of Major A Reade D.S.O. who was soon replaced by Capt PG Sharp. William Marshall, engineer from Bath War Hospital and the Surgical Requisites Association, stayed on. A lady instructor, Miss Anderson, taught basket-making, with the intention of improving dexterity. More motivating was a workshop where amputees made prostheses, and a carpentry workshop to develop woodworking skills. The engineering workshop taught oxy-acetylene welding. Chivers' influence can be recognised in the bookbinding workshop. There was a tailor's shop, a signwriting workshop, a photographic studio, and training in plumbing and shoe mending. The gardens were developed to include a poultry farm and piggery.

By 1924, when the BMA visited Bath for its annual meeting, it was recorded that the *'excellent limb fitting centre supplies the most modern artificial legs, artificial arms being obtained from Roehampton'.*

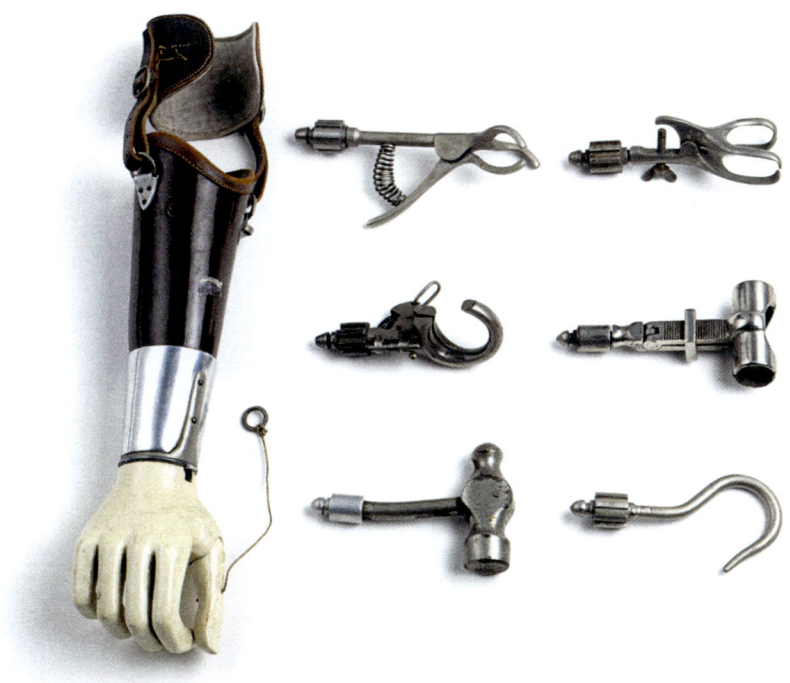

Figure 9.
Lightweight celluloid prosthetic lower arm with workmen's fittings.
Science Museum, London.

Although the number of orthopaedic in-patients was small, this was balanced by a substantial increase in those attending outpatient orthopaedic clinics, responsible for prosthesis fitting and after-care. There were two orthopaedic hubs in the south west, one in Exeter and the other in Bath. The Bath hub was responsible for eleven clinics, which were opened in Bridgewater, Bristol, Chippenham, Dorchester, Glastonbury, Gloucester, Minehead, Swindon, Trowbridge, Taunton, and Yeovil. The availability of the full prosthetics department meant that hand fitments could be tailored to the needs of specific trades. (Figure 9).

By the time of the BMA meeting only 369 beds remained. There were by then no neurology patients left. The five-year average yearly admissions had been one hundred officers and 2,245 other ranks. 4,277 operations had been performed since the Pensions Hospital opened in January 1920. The BMA report mentions the *'particularly good x-ray and physiotherapy departments'*. Radiology had been improved following a specific request from Bath in 1922 for better x-ray equipment. A higher voltage set had been installed for improved thoracic and contrast abdominal radiology. It was one of only three national upgrades at the time, the other two being in the much larger Pensions Hospitals in Leeds and in Liverpool.

The Pensions Hospital closed in December 1928. It had cared for about 15,000 patients. The sixty patients who were still being treated in hospital, a decade after the war ended, were moved to Chepstow. The YMCA hut, erected in October 1917 for recreation and entertainment, was dismantled and re-erected in Locksbrook Road to house the Weston Adult School.

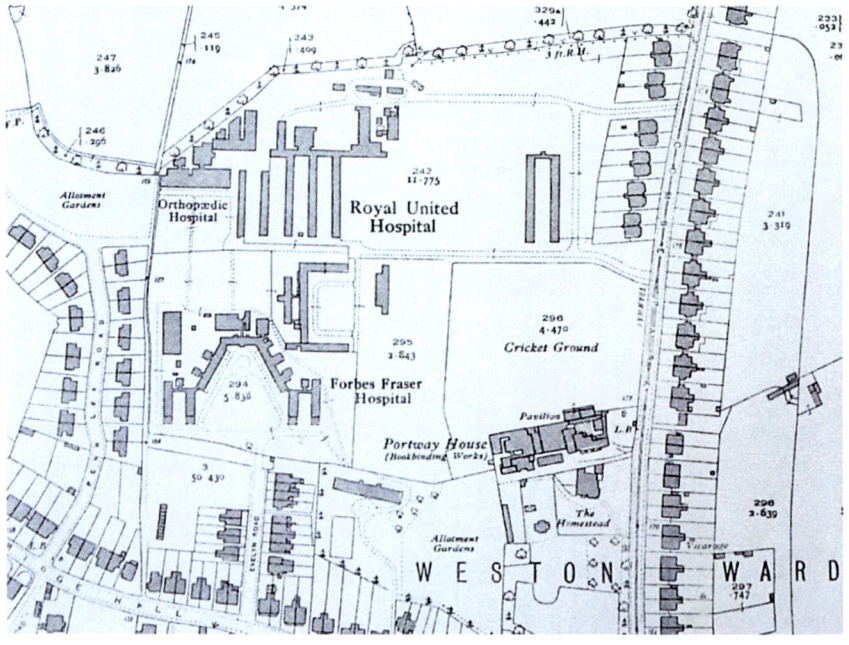

Figure 10. Map showing the hospital site in 1932, with the Pensions Hospital blocks partially dismantled.

Two hospitals remained on the Combe Park site, both opened on 16th May 1924. The planned private hospital had been named the Forbes Fraser Hospital and can be easily seen as the V-shaped building to the south of the picture in figure 10. On the same day the Children's Orthopaedic Hospital was opened, initially with twenty-four beds, eventually expanding to accommodate seventy-two. It was designed with a south-facing terrace for treatment of children in the sun and fresh air.

Of the 90 servicemen buried in Locksbrook Cemetery, at least a quarter died after the Pensions Hospital opened. It is probable that several of these died from the effects of the flu epidemic that swept through the country after the war. The last to be laid to rest was Private H Ridler, of the Royal Army Service Corps, who died on 3rd June 1921, aged fifty-eight.

The vacation of the site set in motion its redevelopment. The temporary wards, erected at the beginning of 1916, were quickly dismantled, leaving only the nurses' accommodation to remain in use for another decade. On 25th October 1930 the foundation stone of the new Royal United Hospital was laid on the Combe Park site. A month before, the foundation stone of the new Bath and Wessex Children's Orthopaedic Hospital was laid. These two events set in train the continuing development of the Combe Park as a hospital, which had started in August 1915 with the preparation of the site for the Bath War Hospital, and continues to this day.

Sources

1. Bath Records Office. Bath War Hospital.
2. National Archives Kew. MH 120/50,52 and 53 and T161/39 and 75
3. Wellcome Library, London 44761i. Physical Therapy at Bath War Hospital. and reverse. Images L 81720 and L 81719.
4. bathwarhospital.org
5. British Library Newspaper archive. Numerous articles in the Bath Chronicle
6. Royal United Hospital NHS Trust. Brownsword Therapies Centre. Bath War Hospital permanent exhibition.
7. Postages H. Physical therapy at Bath War Hospital: Rehabilitation and its links to WWI. JHR. jhrehab.org 01 May 2019.
8. War Graves Commission. Locksbrook Cemetery, Bath

John Dunn (1834 – 1896)
and the Zulu War of 1879

PETER M. DUNN,
MA, MD, FRCP, FRCOG, FRCPCH
Emeritus professor of perinatal medicine and child health, University of Bristol
e-mail: P.M.Dunn@bristol.ac.uk
Presented to the society Monday March 9th 2020

My family, the Dunns, hailed from the Scottish borders. My great, great grandfather, James Dunn was a tailor in Ancrum, Roxboroughshire. Born in 1766, he married Janet Thomson in 1791 and they had a family of six children, four girls and two boys. The eldest boy, my great grandfather, John Adam Dunn, born in 1801, became the toll-master of the bridge over the River Tweed at Kelso. His younger brother, Robert, born in 1804, emigrated from Scotland in 1830.

Incidentally, John and Robert were favourite first names in our family occurring in almost every generation. Indeed my own two sons are named Robert and John ... and true to form John has emigrated.

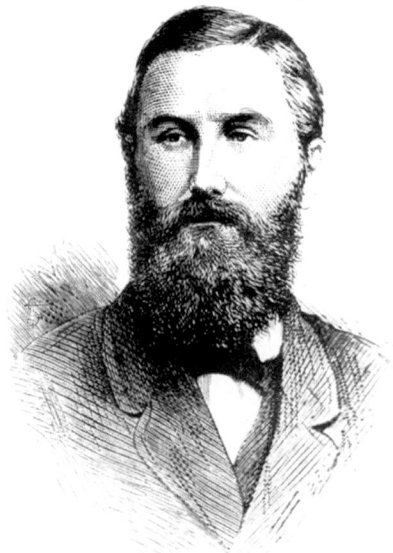

Figure 1. John Dunn (1834 -1896), White Chief of the Zulus

Robert Dunn, at the age of 26, left the shores of Scotland in 1830 to settle in the Eastern Cape, South Africa. There he married Ann Biggar and they had four children, three girls and a boy. The boy, christened John, was born in 1834 soon after the family had moved east along the coast to Port Natal (Figures 1 and 2). There the father, Robert Dunn, thrived as a trader and hunter. He built a store and then in 1839 a substantial dwelling on the ridge overlooking Durban Bay named 'Sea View', along with 2,500 acres of land.

When Robert arrived in Natal there were only about fifty Europeans living there. Some ten years later in 1843 Natal was recognised by Queen Victoria as a colony of the British Empire. By the late 1840s the European population had increased to some 3,000.

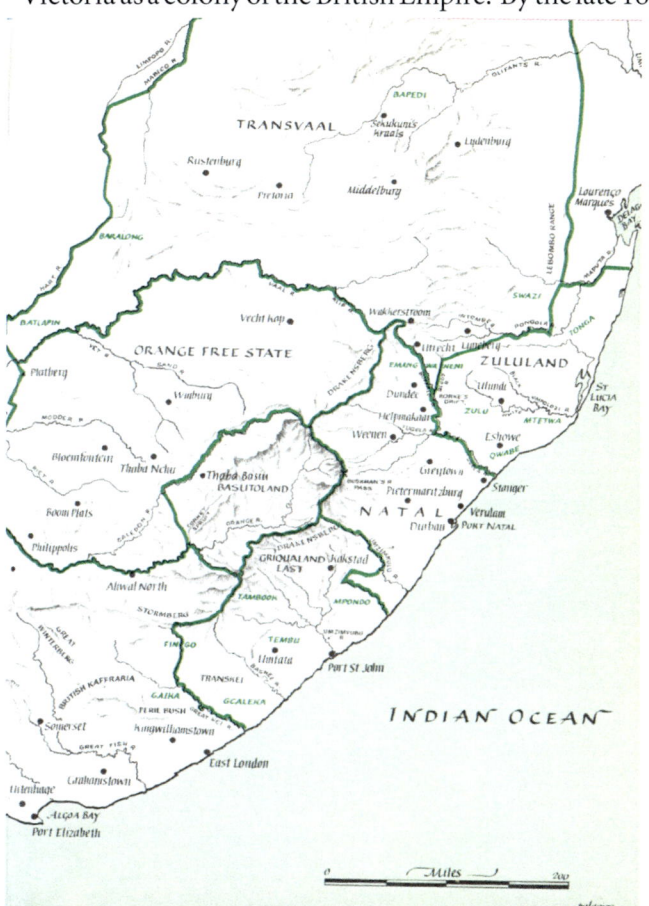

Figure 2: Map of South Africa in 1879

Meanwhile young John Dunn was growing up among the Zulu staff at 'Sea View'. From an early age he was exposed to the Zulu culture and language. Bright, intelligent and quick on the uptake, he had little formal education. His youth was spent in the saddle learning to shoot and to hunt. This not only gave him the opportunity to hone his language skills, but also to observe and accept Zulu customs and social behaviour leading in due course to his acceptance by the Zulus as a 'white Zulu'. They named him 'Jantoni'.

In 1847 John's father, Robert Dunn, was trampled to death by an elephant. 'Sea View' was then sold by his wife Ann and she and her daughters moved back to the East Cape. John, though, aged 14 decided to stay in Natal. He tried his hand as a transport rider but because of his youth was not paid. In disgust he decided to desert the haunts of civilisation for those of large game in Zulu land. So in 1852 at the age of 18 he crossed the Tugela River with his young 15 year old bride, Catherine Pearce, to live among the Zulus. Two years later at the age of 20 he was befriended by, and became assistant to, a retired British Army Captain, Joshua Warmsley. Living with him for the next six years at his home, Nonoti, near the lower drift of the Tugela River, Dunn became thoroughly educated in western ways. There emerged a remarkable combination of a man that could be passed as a Zulu or be entirely at ease in a European environment such as the Durban Club.

At this point it is necessary to digress in order to say a little about the creation of the Zulu nation. In the 18th century as the Europeans, mainly Dutch, were beginning to spread north east from the Cape, Bantu tribes were slowly moving south from Central Africa. At a time when we were engaged in the Napoleonic wars in Europe, a remarkable warrior named Shaka was creating the Zulu nation in the lands to the north and east of Natal (Fig 3).

Though of royal blood Shaka was illegitimate and had had a lonely childhood, being ostracised as he grew up. He was also

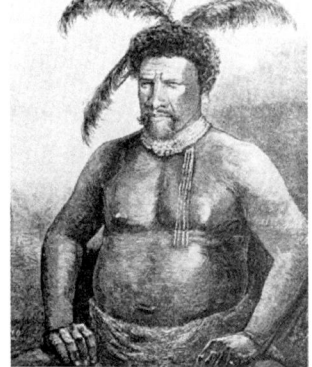

Figure 3: Artist's impression of Shaka, Chief of the Zulus

almost certainly both a homosexual and impotent. He grew to 6'3" and became recognised as a famous warrior not only for his fighting skills but for his tactics in battle. He armed the men of his tribe with short stabbing spears called assegai and drilled them in regiments or impis of around 1,000 men, each with their own traditions, identity and morale (Figs 4 & 5). These Zulus were all extremely fit, capable of covering 50 miles in a day. Gradually Shaka coalesced all the surrounding Bantu tribes by fear and force into a Zulu empire of some two million people,

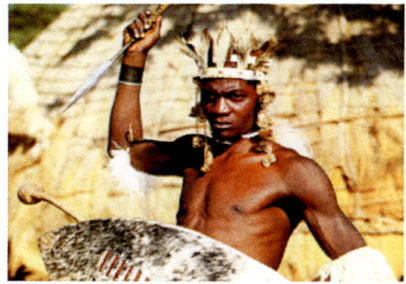

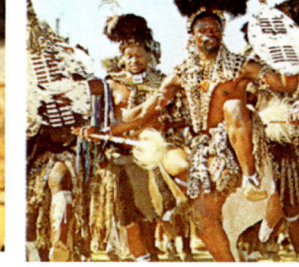

Figure 4: Zulu warrior armed with assegai and shield

Figure 5: Zulus of an impi dancing

settled in an area of land 200 x 100 miles to the north of the Tugela River. Shaka was a fierce despot and a psychopath who ruled by terror. But in 1828 he was assassinated and his brother Dingane then became king. He too, in due course, was assassinated and his place taken by yet another brother, Mpande.

During Mpande's lifetime, two of his sons Cetshwayo and Mbuyasi fought in 1856 for the right to succeed him to the Zulu throne. John gave his support to Mbuyasi and nearly lost his life at the battle of Ndondakuska on the north bank of the Tugela River where Mbuyasi's men were slaughtered to a man.

Notwithstanding, John Dunn turned up at Cetshwayo's kraal the following year, 1857, to request the return of cattle that had been taken by his Zulus after the battle. They belonged to Natal farmers and there was a £250 reward for their recovery. John might have been killed out of hand. Instead Cetshwayo befriended him. As he was to write later: *'I came to love this white man as a brother and made him one of my Indunas, giving him land and wives, daughters of my chiefs.'* (Fig 6) Cetshwayo's support and his subsequent grant of lands between the Tugela and Umlalazi Rivers elevated Dunn into a position of both power and wealth. He assumed the position of both friend and counsellor to Cetshwayo and in 1858 moved permanently into Zululand. In spite of Catherine's objections he married Zulu women from a variety of different clans, always paying the going rate of dowry. He established three main residences on his lands, Mangenthe, Emoyeni and Qwayinduku, together with control of some 6,000 subjects. He never lost the urge to hunt and ivory, hides and skins together with thousands of cattle were the main source of his income (Fig 7).

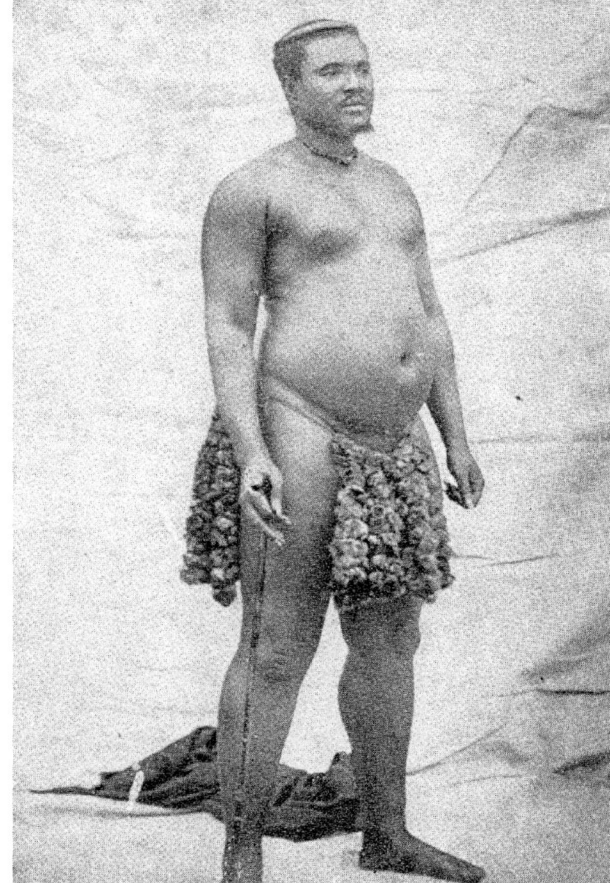

Figure 6: Cetshwayo (1827-1884), King of the Zulus

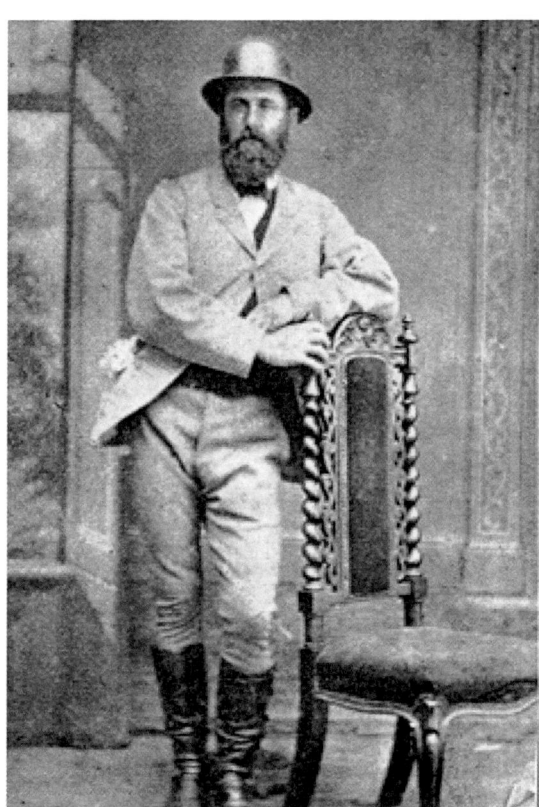

Fig 7: John Dunn (Jantoni) (1834-1896) in the 1850s

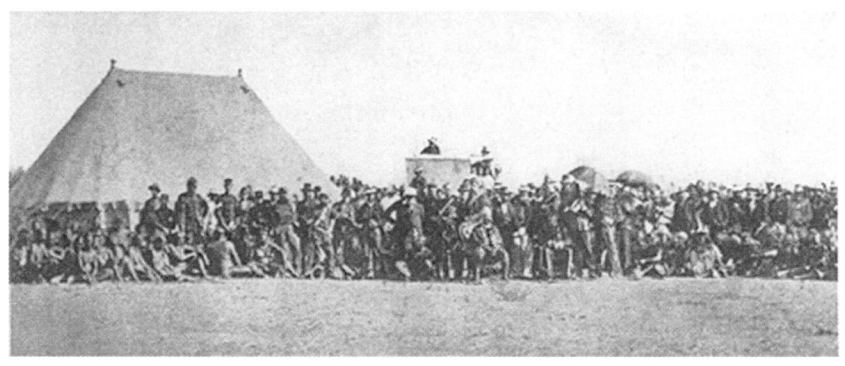

Figure 8: King Cetshwayo's coronation, 1873

In 1873 Mpande died at the age of 45 and Cetshwayo was crowned King of the Zulus (Fig 8), the ceremony being attended by Theophilus Shepstone, Secretary for Native Affairs in Natal (Fig 9).
John Dunn was also there and gave Cetshwayo a fine carriage drawn by white horses (Fig 10).
Cetshwayo was a tall, muscular man with finely chiselled features and a regal and dignified air. With the advice of John Dunn, he was careful not to quarrel with the British in Natal though he was in dispute with Boer farmers who were making inroads into his lands in the north-west. Still, the British were understandably anxious at having a warrior nation with an army of 50 impis on its borders. Nor was the situation made easier by the fact that Cetshwayo imported some fifteen thousand rifles into Zululand soon after coming to the throne.

Sir Bartle Frere, High Commissioner for South Africa (Fig 11), decided to settle the matter out of hand. He mobilised an army of some three thousand or more troops, half of them British, under Major General Thesiger, Baron Chelmsford (Fig 12), and issued an ultimatum to Cetshwayo which virtually amounted to the surrender of his nation. Among his demands were that Cetshwayo's army was to be disarmed and disbanded and that a British diplomatic resident was to be appointed to settle any future disputes between the Europeans and Zulus.

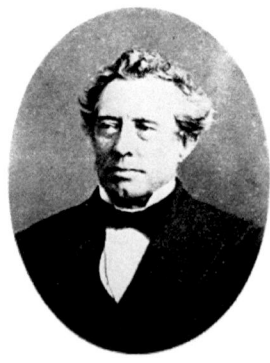

Figure 9: Theophilus Shepstone, Secretary for Native Affairs in Natal

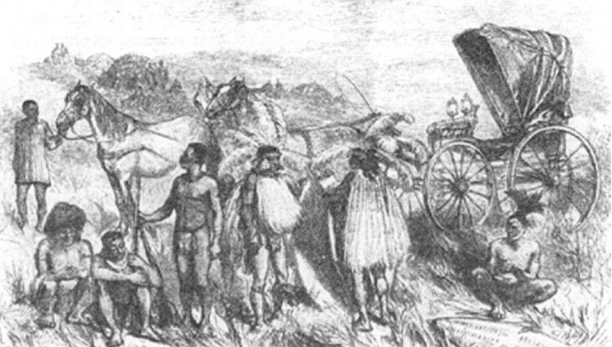

Fig 10: John Dunn's coronation present to Cetshwayo

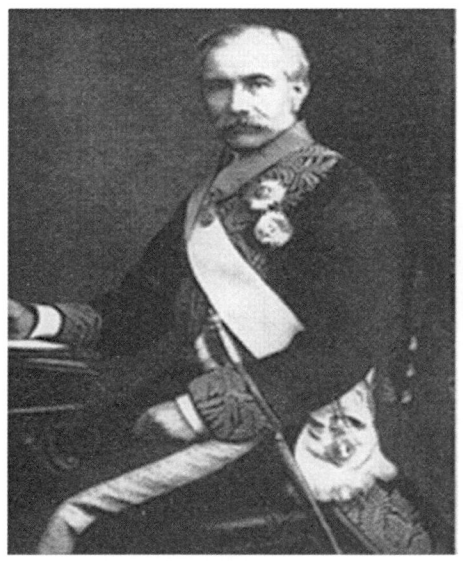
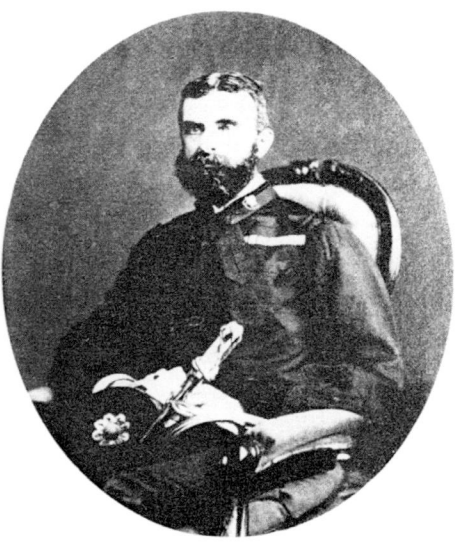

Fig 11: Sir Bartle Frere (1815-1884), High Commissioner for South Africa

Fig 12: General Thesiger, Baron Chelmsford (1827-1905)

Furthermore, he gave Cetshwayo no time to negotiate the matter. It was a truly disgraceful performance for which the High Commissioner was later severely reprimanded by the British Government. Three weeks later on January 2nd 1879, Chelmsford invaded Zululand across the Buffalo River at Rorke's Drift with his main force of around two thousand troops, mainly European.

The outbreak of war faced John Dunn with an acute dilemma (Fig 13). He wished to remain neutral but this was not permitted by Chelmsford. So prior to the outbreak of hostilities he moved his family and some 2,000 of his followers together with 3,000 head of cattle across the lower drift of the Tugela River into Natal. At this, Cetshwayo, feeling betrayed, sent an impi to destroy John's residences in Zululand. Sadly, in the flames, the history of the Zulu nation that Dunn had been writing was lost for good.

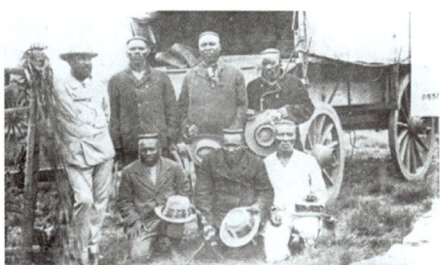

Fig 13: Chief John Dunn with his indunas, 1879

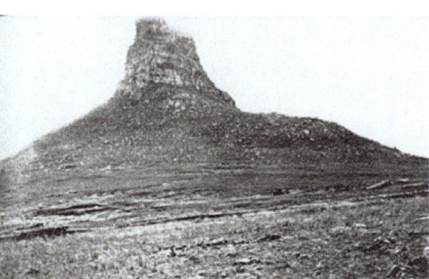

Fig 14: Isandhlwana, January 1879

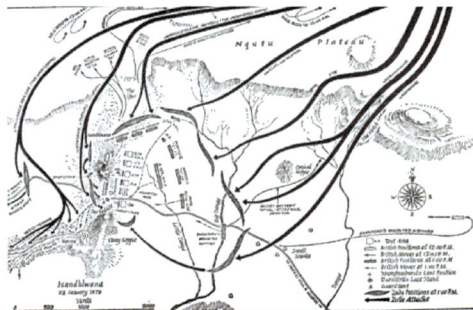

Fig 15: Cetshwayo's impis attack on the British camp at Isandhlwana, January 1879

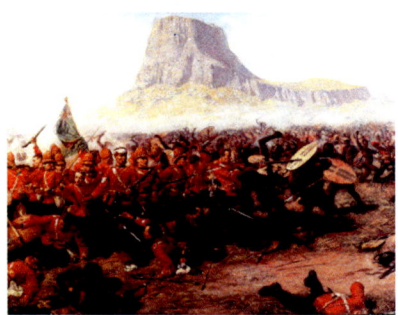

Fig 16: The battle of Isandhlwana where 900 British troops were slaughtered by the Zulus

After eighteen days, the British force had established camp at Isandhlwana, a rock crowned hill, ten miles into Zululand (Fig 14). The going was very difficult with no roads for the many hundreds of cattle-drawn wagons. On January 21st, Chelmsford, with some four hundred mounted men, rode forward eight miles to reconnoitre the next camp site. While he was absent, twenty of Cetshwayo's impis, some twenty thousand men, descended on Isandhwana (Fig 15). At this many of the native troops panicked and fled. The British formed up and fought until they had expended all their fifty rounds each of ammunition. Unfortunately, the reserve rounds were stored in screwed down wooden crates and there was a problem finding the screwdrivers. In the end, all nine hundred British troops were overwhelmed and killed (Fig 16). Before they died, though, about two thousand Zulus had been slain and many more wounded.

Meanwhile, Cetshwayo's brother, Dabulamanzi (Fig 17), with three Impis, had bypassed Isandhlwana and attacked the company of British troops defending Rorke's Drift (Fig 18).

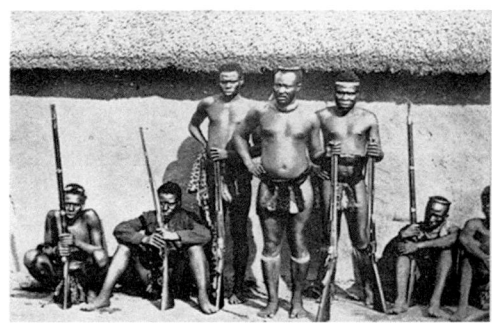

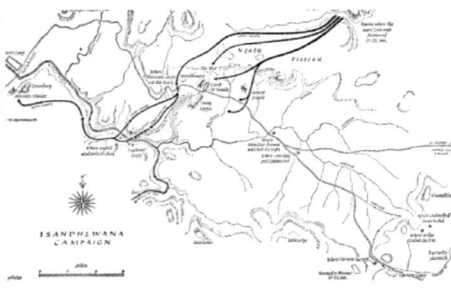

Figure 17: Dabulamanzi, Cetshwayo's half-brother, who led the attack on Rorke's Drift.

Fig 18: The Zulu impis attack on Rorke's Drift, January 1879

After fierce fighting they were repulsed with a loss of another one thousand Zulus by the men of B Company of the 2nd/24th commanded by Bromhead and Chard (Figs 19 & 20). Both Bromhead and Chard and nine others were subsequently awarded the Victoria Cross.

Chelmsford had presided over the greatest defeat sustained by the British army in Victorian times. He had underestimated the Zulu threat and had failed to laager the camp at Isandhlwana or to leave clear instructions for its defence.

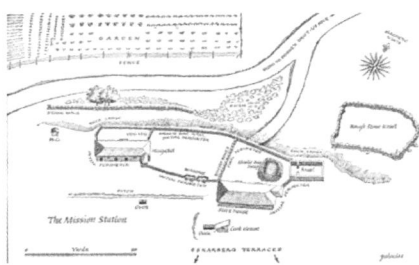

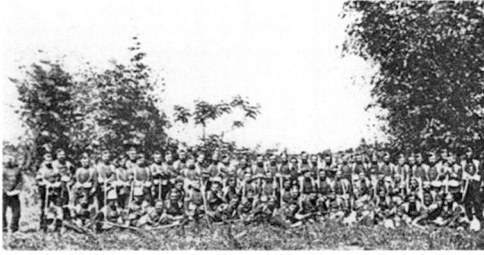

Figure 19:
The Mission Station at Rorke's Drift

Figure 20: The men of B Company of the 2nd/24th that successfully defended the Mission Station at Rorke's Drift

In his absence the British attempted to defend too large an area instead of concentrating their troops in a tight formation against the hillside. In Britain the news contributed to the fall of Disraeli's government. It also led to a public outcry and to the dispatch of some 16,000 troops (Fig 21) accompanied by Gatling guns (Fig 22), field guns and no less than four generals. Meanwhile, Chelmsford was desperate to re-establish his reputation by achieving a victory over the Zulus before Sir Garnett Wolseley, one of the four generals, took over as commander-in-chief.

Chelmsford organised his forces into two columns (Fig 23). The first and smaller one under the command of General Crealock were to cross the Tugela River at the lower drift and advance towards Ulundi, Cetshwayo's main karal, some seventy-five miles away. His force was accompanied by John Dunn as Political and Intelligence Officer. While this column made some progress reaching Eshowe twenty miles into Zululand and winning an encounter with the Zulus at the battle of Gingindhlovu on the way, its progress was very slow.

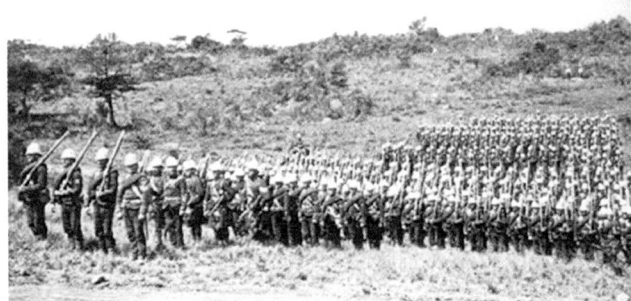

Fig 21: Some of the reinforcements despatched from England following the defeat at Isandlhwana

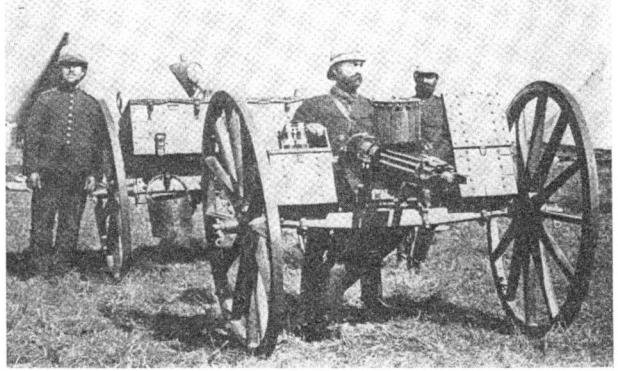

Fig 22: A Gattling gun used during the second invasion of Zululand

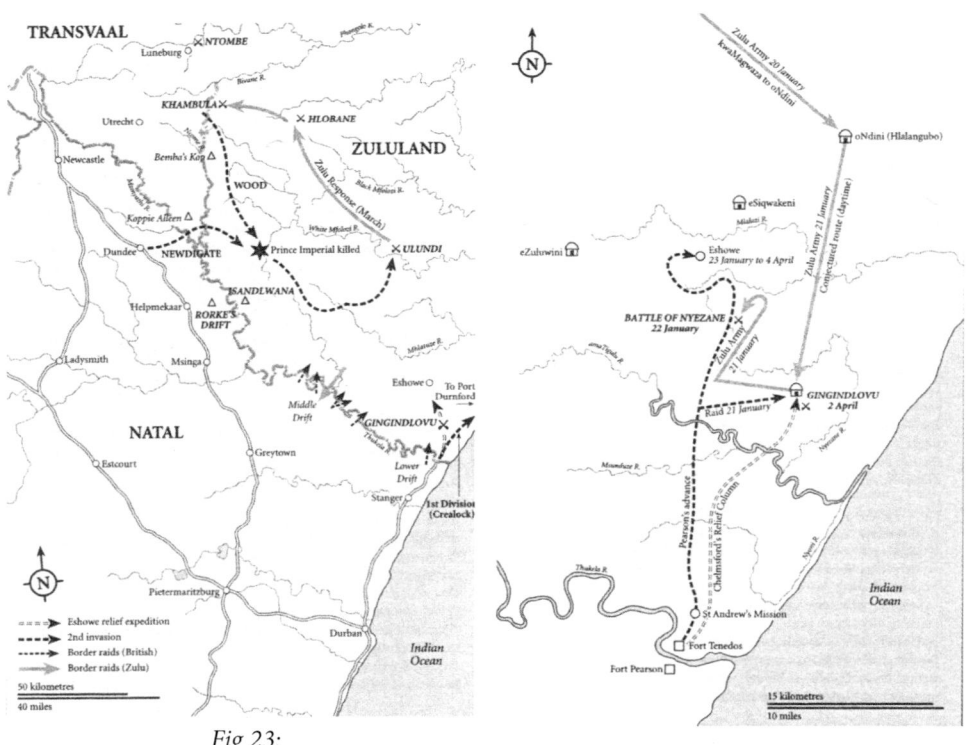

Fig 23:
Track of General Crealock's first column of the second invasion of Zululand

Fig 24:
Track of Lord Chelmsford's second column invading Zululand in 1879

Meanwhile the main invasion force of approximately twenty-three thousand troops under Chelmsford crossed the Buffalo River at Landsman's Drift, fifteen miles north of Rorke's Drift on May 16th (Figure 24). Accompanied by seven hundred wagons pulled by 12,000 oxen over rough ground without roads, progress was again slow but by the beginning of July the column had reached the White Umfolozi River, four miles from Ulundi, Cetshwayo's royal kraal.

Meanwhile, Sir Garnett Wolseley had landed in Durban on 28th June and immediately fired off instructions to Chelmsford to hold everything until he arrived up-country. But there was no holding Chelmsford. On July 4th, his forces crossed the Umfolozi. The Zulus attacked with

their usual courage but were slaughtered in the Battle of Ulundi (Fig 25), none getting within thirty yards of the British defensive square.
So Chelmsford achieved his victory though he had to outwit both Sir Garnett and Cetshwayo to get it. The Zulu monarch had never wanted the war. He was genuinely bewildered by the nature of the issues at stake. The terms of the ultimatum had been completely impossible and he had been invaded before he could discuss conditions or indeed comply with them. He had simply sent his impis in the direction of the invading column and the results of the battles at Isandhwana and Rorke's Drift had appalled him. The Zulu losses had been tremendous. All he wished to know was what were the terms needed to halt the war. However, his approaches to Chelmsford were either disbelieved or disregarded.

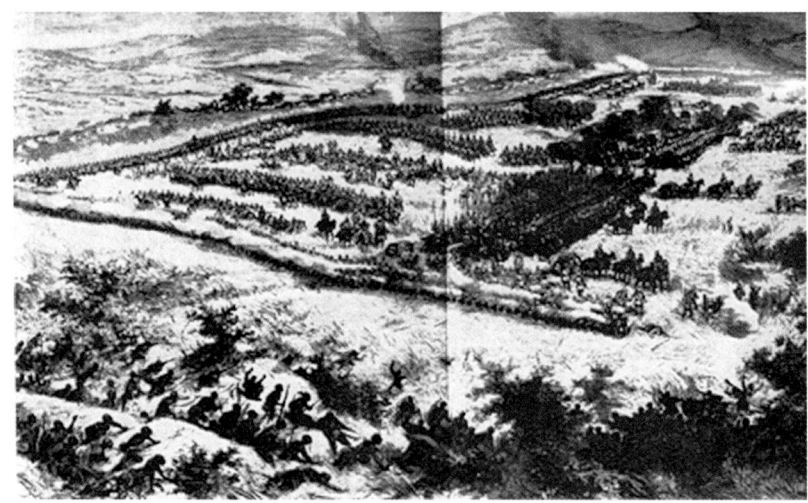

Fig 25: The British square at the Battle of Ulundi, July 4th 1879

With his victory and the burning of Ulundi (Fig 26), Chelmsford was happy to leave whatever remained of the Zulu campaign to Wolseley. He returned to Britain where Queen Victoria invited him to Balmoral and made him a Knight, Grand Cross of the Order of the Bath. Furthermore, he was promoted to Lieutenant General in 1882 and to full General in 1884.

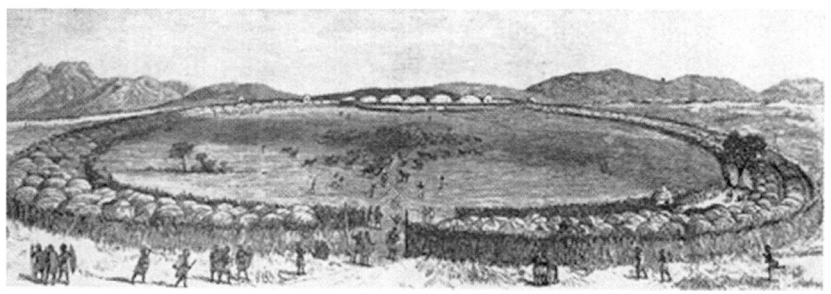

Figure 26: The Royal Craal of Ulundi

Sir Garnett's laconic comment was: *'He is a very nice fellow but Lord forbid he should ever command troops in the field'.* Chelmsford died in 1905 at the age of seventy-eight.

The day before the battle Cetshwayo had left Ulundi. Eventually he was tracked down and on September 7th was taken as a prisoner to Durban and then on to Cape Town (Fig 27). He was 52 years old. Instead of appearing a fierce warrior, he seemed to the people he met to be both gentle and regal. As he said: *'I am only a child and the British government is my father'.* In 1882, dressed in European clothes, he was taken to England (Fig 28).

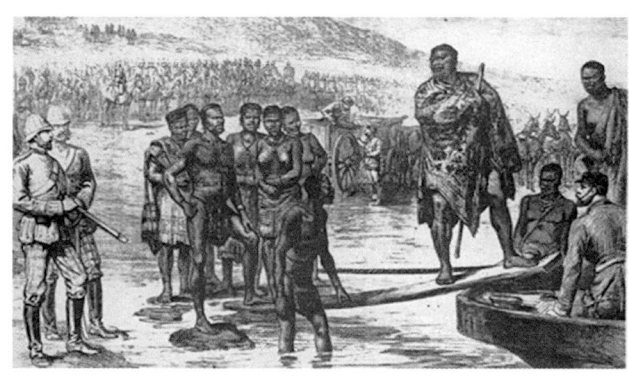

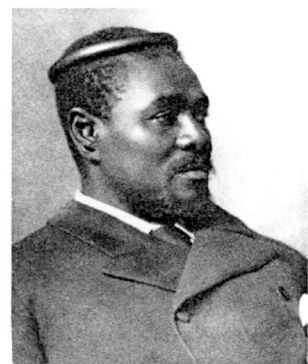

Figure 27: Cetshwayo leaving Natal as a prisoner

Fig 28: Cetshwayo, King of the Zulus in European clothes

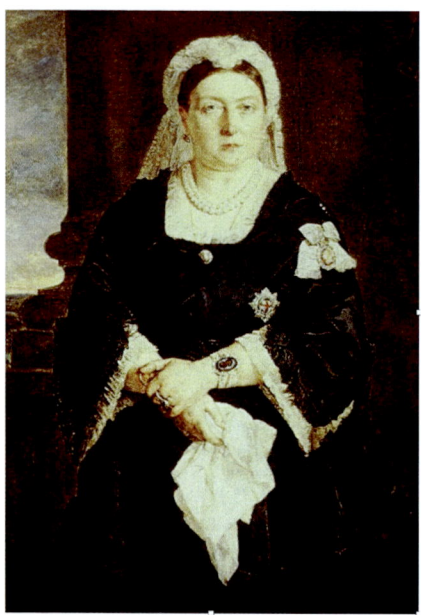
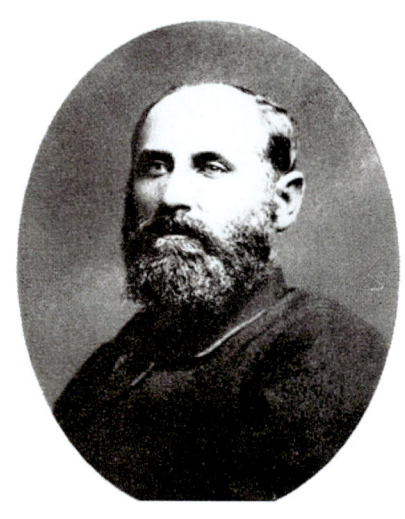

Figure 29: Queen Victoria

Fig 30: John Dunn (Jantoni), White Chief of the Zulus

There he was greeted as a noble and popular figure who had been badly wronged. Queen Victoria invited him to lunch at Osbourne (Fig 28). In 1883 he was returned to Zululand as a minor chief but with little power or authority and the following year he died.

The 1879 war with the Zulus had cost Britain the sum of £5,230,000. Of the 32,000 men who had taken to the field, seventy-six officers and 1,007 men had lost their lives while another thirty-seven officers and 206 men had been wounded. In addition seventeen officers and 330 men had died of disease.

On July 7th, 1879, three days after the battle of Ulundi, Major General Crealock wrote formally to Sir Garnett, the new Commander in Chief, to draw attention to the invaluable services performed by Mr. John Dunn, attached to him as Political and Intelligence Officer (Fig 30). He wrote:

'It's impossible for me to exaggerate the useful information obtained by this officer, not only for me but also for Lord Chelmsford. His great

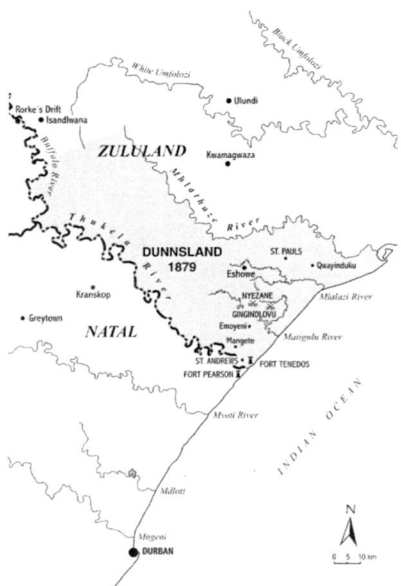

Figure 31: Dunnsland, to the east of the Tugela River, 1879

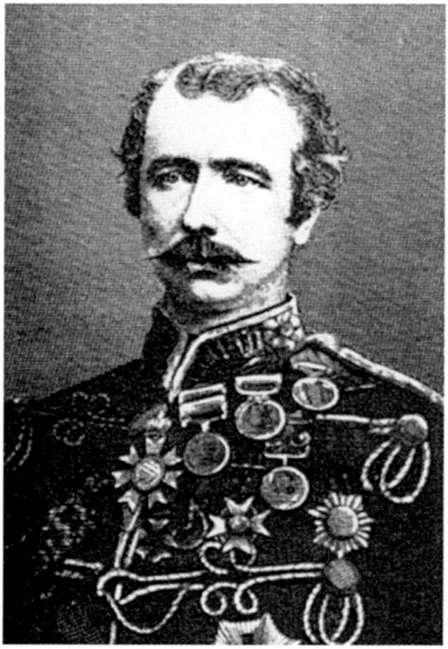

Figure 32: Sir Garnett Wolseley, 1833-1913

knowledge of this country and of its people, his long residence in it, and the perfect confidence evidently reposed in him by all classes of Zulus, have not only been most useful to me from a military point of view, but have also undoubtedly tended more than anything else to bringing about the satisfactory condition of things which I have already had occasion to report to His Excellency, namely the submission of many influential Chiefs of this District, with their families and followers, and their cattle. I have found his local information regarding roads, rivers and natural obstacles, remarkably accurate, and of the greatest service. I have found him perfectly reliable and perfectly trustworthy, and silence and discretion itself, and I cannot too strongly recommend him to the favour of His Excellency'.

As a result of his services Queen Victoria, through Wolseley, awarded John Dunn (Fig 31) a block of land beyond the Tugela and Buffalo Rivers, stretching forty miles north along the coast and eighty miles inland, twice the size of the land originally given to him by Cetshwayo. There John Dunn settled and lived in great style as the White Chief of the Zulus together with his own large family, the natives of his Dunn clan and his cattle. It became known as Dunnsland.

Following his arrival, Sir Garnett Wolseley (Fig 32) set about disarming and pacifying the Zulu clans. While he may have been a great General he was certainly no administrator. Instead of annexing Zululand, he divided it up into twelve small kingdoms in addition to Dunnsland, each with their own Zulu chief. At the same time he appointed a British resident at Eshowe in Dunnsland to keep order and settle disputes. Alas, he failed to provide the resident with the power to achieve this and Zululand soon lapsed into unrest, chaos and disorder. Twenty years later in 1902, Zululand was opened to European settlement.

In 1894 John Dunn's eyesight began to fail and in 1896, after a brief illness, he died of dropsy and heart failure at his Emoyeni home. Aged 61, he was mourned by his 49 wives and 116 children (Fig 33). Undoubtedly he was one of the most powerful and influential characters of Zululand in the 19th century.

During the 20th century, Dunnsland was steadily eroded until with Apartheid it finally ceased to be. Some of Jantoni's children had married Europeans while others had merged into the Zulu native population. All, however, remained proud of their clan and the thriving Dunns Descendants Association. A visit to Jantoni's well-kept grave, lovingly attended, reflected on the high esteem in which this extraordinary 'White Zulu Chief' had been and still is held (Fig 34).

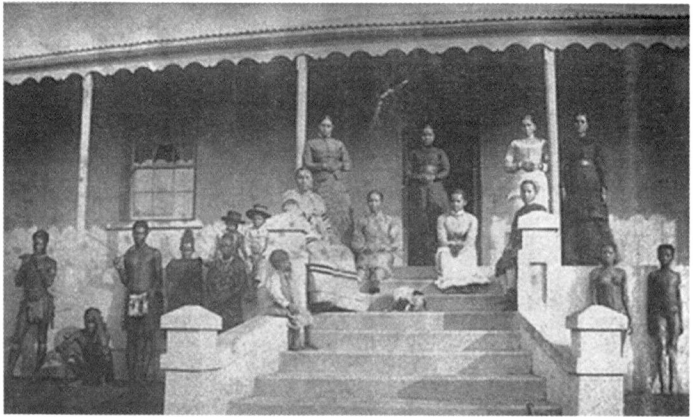

Figure 33: Catherine Dunn with some of her children at their homestead

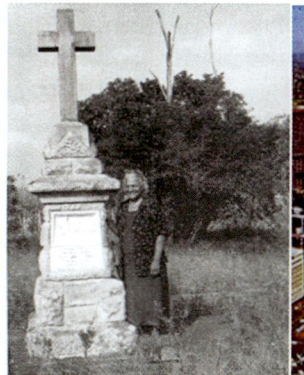 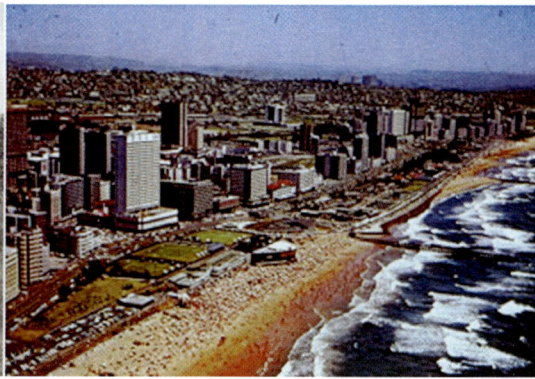

Figure 34: John Dunn's grave erected in 1920

Figure 35: Durban, Natal, 1979

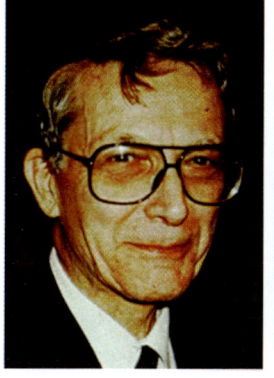 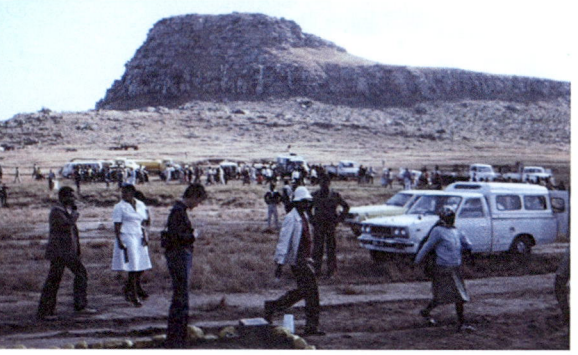

Figure 36:
Dr. Walter Loening,
University of Durban

Figure 37:
Centenary celebrations at Isandhlwana,
May 25th, 1979

In 1979 I was invited to speak at a perinatal conference in Durban, Natal (Fig 35). I was met there by Walter Loening, a senior lecturer in the University of Natal's department of paediatrics (Fig 36).

He mentioned to me that the following day he was going to attend the Zulu Centenary celebration of their defeat of the British army at Isandhlwana in 1879. Would I like to come? Would I not! So 5am the next morning found us on our way driving one hundred miles north into KwaZulu. By the time we arrived in Isandhlwana the celebrations were in full swing (Fig 37).

Many hundreds of Zulu warriors had congregated in groups, often on little hillocks (Fig 38). Every now and then, a fully kitted warrior would get to his feet, disclaim on the greatness of his race and achievements, all the time stamping his feet and working himself into a passion of excitement. He would then charge down the hillock towards the onlookers waving his weapon over his head (Fig 39). Naturally I was keen to record the action with my little camera. As I focused the viewfinder a knobkerrie whistled over my head. Werner promptly dragged me away: *'You don't know how nearly you had your brains dashed out'*, he told me.

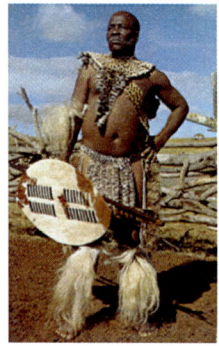

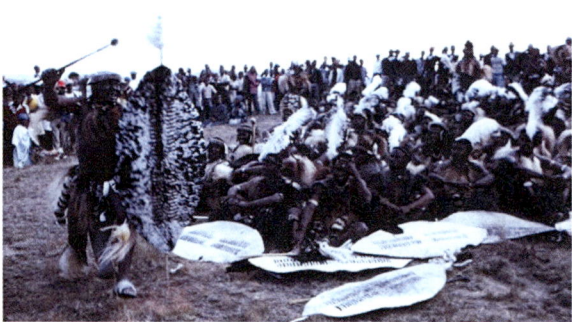

Figure 38:
Zulu warrior, 1979

Figure 39: Zulu warrior with knobkerrie breaks away from his group (see text)

But it was a wonderful occasion. The Zulu womenfolk (Figs 40 & 41) had also turned out in great numbers, all decked out in their best native costumes. I also bumped into Chief Butelezi and King Goodwill Zulu (Fig 42).

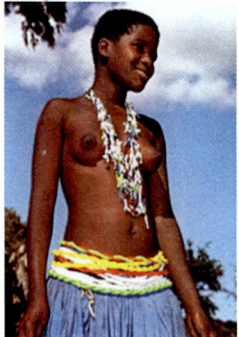

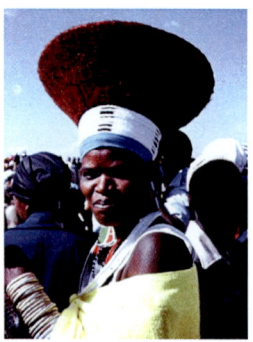

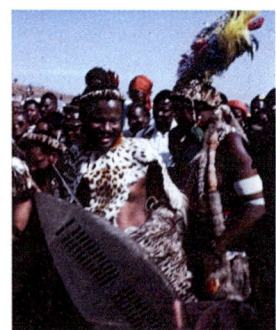

Figure 40:
Zulu maiden

Figure 41:
A Zulu matron

Fig 42: Chief Buthelazi and King Goodwill Zulu at Isandhlwana, May 25th, 1979

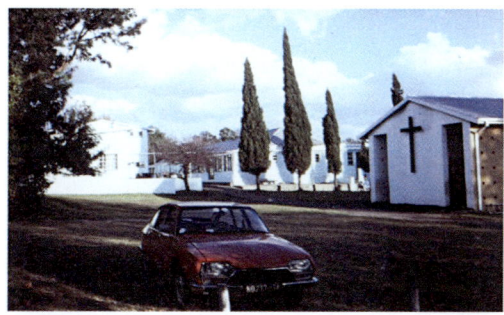

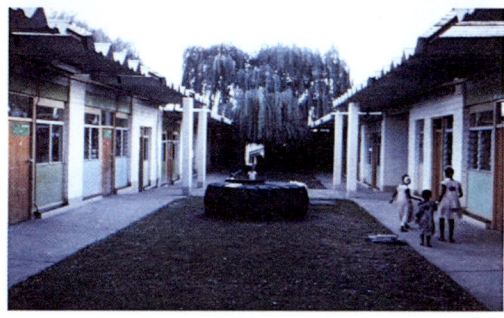

*Figures 43 and 44:
Charles Johnson Memorial
Hospital, KwaZulu*

All too soon it was time to return to Durban. I was sad not to have had the opportunity to also visit Rorke's Drift, some ten miles away but I did manage to visit the Charles Johnson Memorial Hospital in KuaZulu (Fig 43). This hospital of 500 beds had been founded in 1945 and was run by European medical volunteers (Fig 44). I was especially interested as my nephew, Dr. James Stuart, had worked there for a year in 1977. His father, Dr. Jack Stuart, had also spent some months there. A few years later in 1986 yet another nephew, my godson, Dr. Richard Garratt, served there as senior surgeon for 12 years.

While at the Charles Johnson Memorial Hospital Richard, my nephew, fell in love with a Zulu nurse, Nomthandaze, which means 'daughter of prayer'. She was also known by the shorter nickname, Thandi. In 1992 they decided to get married back in England in Warminster, Wiltshire (Fig 45). As her father was in South Africa, I, as uncle and godfather, was invited to give her away and also to speak at the celebration dinner afterwards.

Shortly before the wedding, I had learnt to my surprise that Thandi was a member of the Dunn clan which was still thriving in Natal.

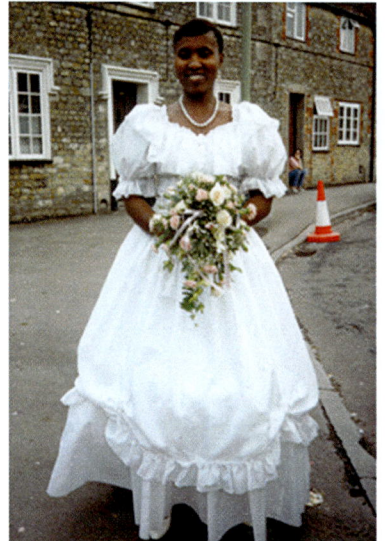 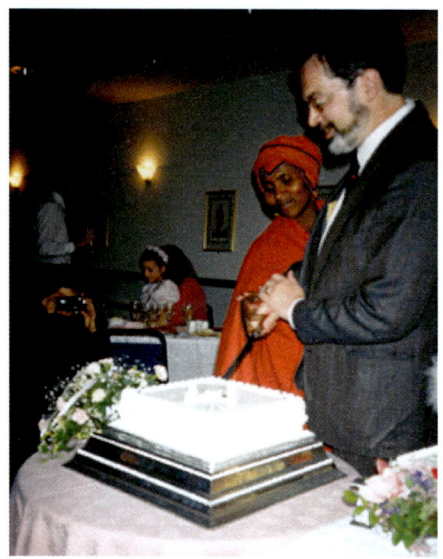

Fig 45: Thandi Dunn before her wedding in Warminster, 1992

Fig 46: Dr. Richard Garratt with his bride, Thandi, cutting their wedding cake, 1992

Indeed, Jantoni's last wife, Noyintaba, had only died in the early 1970s at the age of ninety-eight. I should also mention that following the end of Apartheid the Dunn clan had successfully sued the South African government for the return of their lands which had been confiscated earlier. All this gave me the main focus for my speech. I told the story of my great-grand-uncle, Robert Dunn, emigrating from Scotland in 1830 and then the story of his son, Jantoni, as the White Chief of Zululand, ending by saying that it was possible that Richard and Thandi may indeed have shared a great, great, great grandfather (Fig 46).

It was a good tale and went down well. Alas, my story got back to the Thandi's family in KwaZulu where it led to concern about consanguinity and whether the marriage should be allowed to go ahead. Fortunately, all was well and the happy couple duly married a second time in Natal in Zulu dress and with the roasting of an ox.

****

Envoi

When I had spoken about John Dunn, 'Jantoni', at Richard and Thandi's wedding I believed, but was not certain, that my great grand-uncle, Robert Dunn, was the same man as the father of Jantoni, White Chief of the Zulus. Since then I have done more research. Though both men emigrated from Scotland at the same time, Jantoni's father had come from Inverness while my great grand-uncle had left the Scottish Borders. Somewhat sadly, I have to admit that they were not in fact the same person.

Bibliography

1. Dunn, J. John Dunn, Cetywayo, and the three generals. Ed. by D.C.F. Moore. Pietermaritzburg, Natal, May 1886. Publ. By the Natal Printing and Publishing Co.
2. Elliott, Aubrey. Sons of Zulu. Collins, London, 1978.
3. Knight, Ian. The National Army Museum Book of the Zulu War. Pan Macmillan Books Ltd., London, 2003.
4. KönigKrämer, A., Lock, R. and Quantrill, P. Foreword to John Dunn, Cetywayo and the three generals, 1886. Durban, KwaZulu-Natal, 2006.
5. Lock, Ron. Zulu Conquered. The March of the Red Soldiers, 1828-1884. Frontline Books, London, 2010.
6. Morris, D.R. The washing of the Spears. Publ. Jonathan Cape, London, 1966.
7. Taylor, Stephen. Shaka's Children. A history of the Zulu people. Harper Collins Publ., London, 1995.

Shaking Hands With the King of the Zulus
Editor's Note

P. GODDARD

As I sat listening to Peter Dunn's talk about the Zulu War I felt the stirring of a memory. I recalled conversations that my brother and I had enjoyed over supper with my grandmother, when she was living with us in South Croydon in the 1960s. There was a dim recollection that she had told us that she had actually met the King of the Zulus. I dismissed this at first but the next day I telephoned my brother to ask whether he remembered the conversations. Unfortunately he did not and I thought that was the end of the matter. Several days later I chanced upon some correspondence from my Grandmother and to my surprise this confirmed my recollection.

My grandmother, Florence Goddard (née Brown) wrote a letter in 1976 to her grandchildren. Born in 1880, at the time of writing the letter she was almost 96. The 4th side is reproduced on the next page and states:

'Of course the Zulu (war) was before I was born and Queen Victoria invited Cetewayo to come to England and he accepted with his kraal and encamped in the grounds of Crystal Palace. The camp was surrounded by thick white ropes.

At one corner of the camp Cetewayo used to come and liked to shake hands with anyone who would come there.

One day, and I expect it must be my very earliest memories, my father and mother (and I expect my sister) went to the Crystal Palace and my father carrying me I think put me down in front of a Big Black man for him to shake my hand.

I grew up with the knowledge that I had shaken hands with the chief of the Zulus'.

Of course the Zulu war was before I was born & Queen Victoria invited Cetewayo to come to England & he accepted & came with his kraal & encamped in the grounds of the Crystal Palace. The camp was ~~suggested~~ surrounded by thick white ropes.

At one corner of the camp Cetewayo used to come & liked to shake hands with anyone who would come there.

One day & I ~~expect~~ it must be my very ~~earliest~~ memories my father & mother (& I expect my sister) went to the Crystal Palace & my father carrying me I think put me down in front ~~of~~ a Big Black man for him to shake my hand & grew up with the knowledge that I had shaken hands with the Chief of the Zulus.

*Letter by Florence Goddard (née Brown) written in 1976 when she was nearly 96
The letter describes how she met the king of the Zulus!*

The History of the Victoria Cross
Medical VCs, Harold Ackroyd and other VC Heroes.
CHRIS ACKROYD

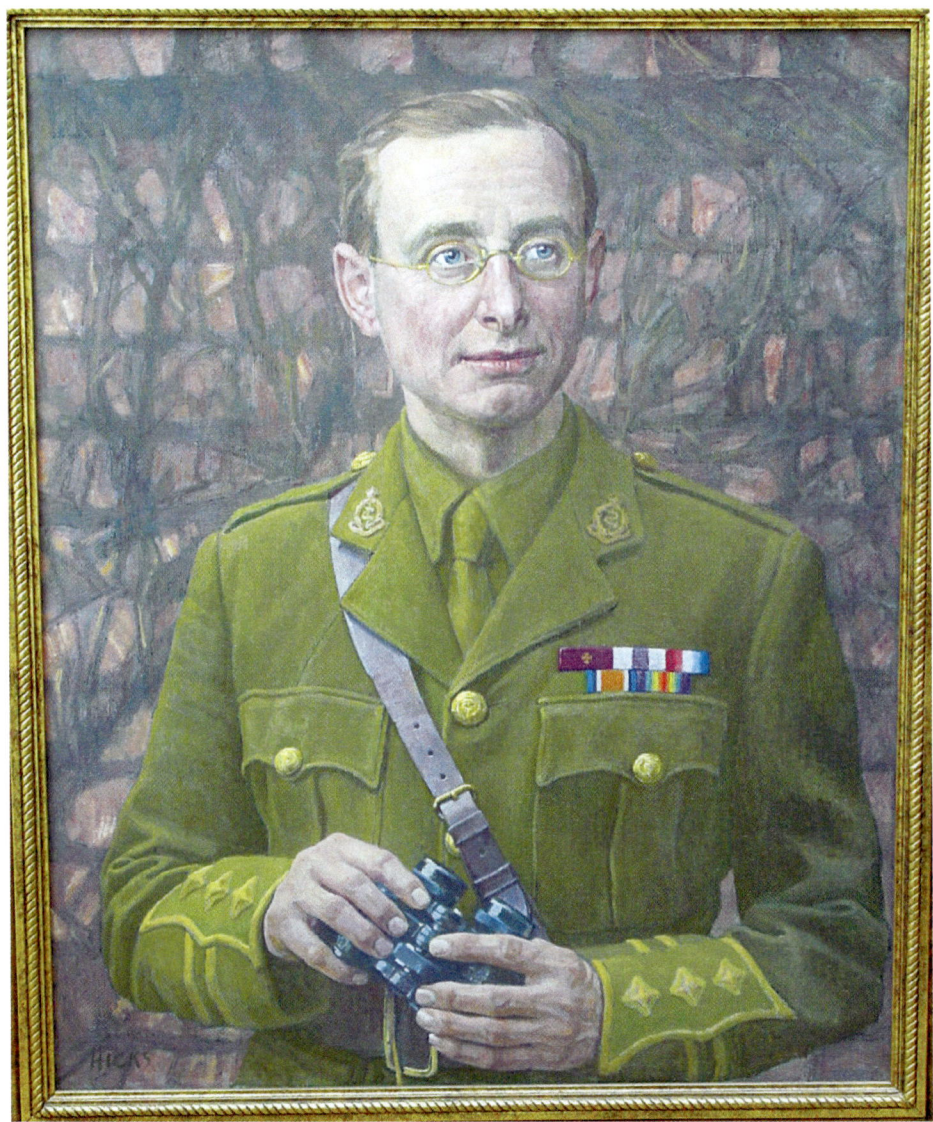

Harold by J Hicks

It is 103 years since my grandfather Capt. Harold Ackroyd was awarded the Victoria Cross while rescuing wounded soldiers from no-man's-land at the beginning of the third Battle of Ypres, Passchendaele, in August 1917. The Victoria Cross was founded by Queen Victoria in 1856 after the 1st Crimea war and is the highest national award for valour. The award has been made to 1,359 individuals and three people have had the award for a second time. The medals are struck from the cascabals of Chinese cannons probably captured from the Russians in the Crimea.

The first VC was awarded to Midshipman Charles Lucas in 1856 in the Baltic and the most recent to LCpl. Joshua Leakey in 2015 in Afghanistan. There are nine living award holders. There have been forty-four awards made to forty-two Medical Staff and of particular interest are the double award holders Lt Col. Arthur Martin-Leake, and Capt. Noel Chavasse both young medical officers in the Boer War and WWI who on numerous occasions rescued injured soldiers while under fire. Lt Col. Ferdinand Le Quesne VC, a Jersey man, was a medical officer who in 1889 in Burma was awarded the Cross after rescuing fellow soldiers while under fire. He died in 1950 and was buried in Canford Cemetery Bristol and he left his medals to the Societe Jersiaise Museum.

Harold Ackroyd was born in Southport in 1877, the second son of a taylor and draper. The family fortunes changed when his mother inherited a sizable sum from her father, a cotton waste dealer in Bolton. After his early schooling, he attended Shrewsbury School and from there gained admission to Gonville and Caius College Cambridge. Harold qualified in medicine at Guy's Hospital in 1904. His career progressed and he moved back to Cambridge as a research scientist, where he met his future wife, Mabel Smythe who was Matron of the Strangeways Research Hospital. In 1908 Harold was awarded a BMA scholarship which he held for three years and he continued a research career at Cambridge. He published at least six papers on Purine metabolism. The last in 1916 was co-authored with Sir Frederick Gowland Hopkins who became the first Professor of Biochemistry.

The first World War was declared on 4th August 1914. Six months later recruitment was at fever pitch and Harold, although aged

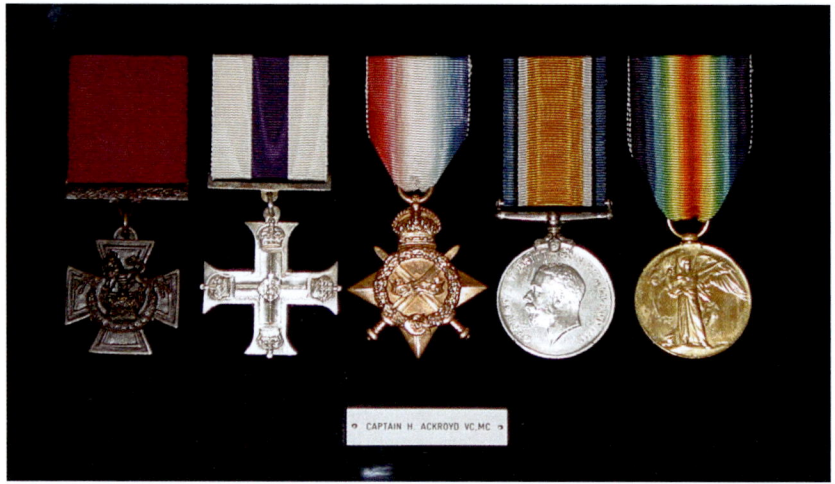

Harold's medals

thirty-seven years and with no recent medical experience, volunteered to join up and was attached to the Royal Berkshire Regiment. After initial training, in July 1915 they were transported over to France to prepare for the great battle of the Somme in the summer of 1916. It was there in mid July that he was involved in the the bloody battle to secure Delville Wood. As a result of his actions to rescue more than a thousand casualties he received eleven recommendations for the Victoria Cross, but was awarded the Military Cross in October 1916.

In November the Regiment moved up to Ypres to prepare for the battle of Passchendaele in July 1917. It was here on 31st July and 1st August that the Regiment was involved in vicious fighting east of Ypres trying to secure Glencorse Wood. At the end of the action Harold had received no less than twenty-three separate recommendations for the Victoria Cross and this award was announced in the London Gazette on 6th September. In the continued fighting in the days that followed, on 11th August, Harold was caught in a shell hole tending the wounded in no-man's-Land, he stood up to signal to the stretcher bearers. He was shot through the head by a sniper's bullet and died instantly.

I inherited the full set of Harold's medals from my Father in 1988, the Victoria Cross, the Military Cross, and the three campaign medals. After 15 years and much debate within the family I finally decided that the best thing would be to sell the medals and realise their value

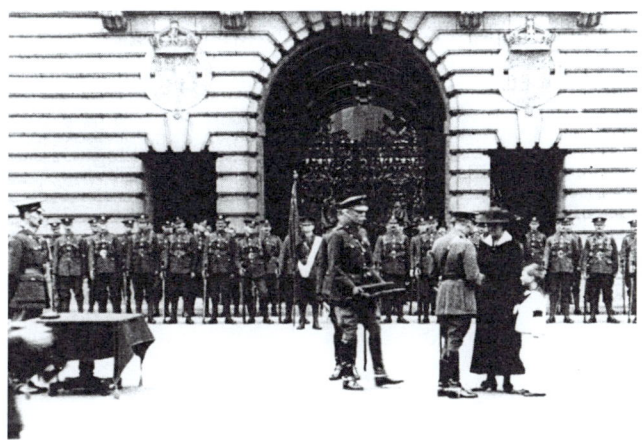

Investiture Photo of Mabel & Stephen with HRH George V

to enable us to endow a medical scholarship at Harold's Cambridge College, Gonville and Caius. After a cloak and dagger sale we now know that the medals were bought by Lord Ashcroft for his collection of over 250 VC`s and GCs, the largest collection in the world. The collection is now on display in the Lord Ashcroft Gallery at the Imperial War Museum. The gallery was opened by the Princess Royal in November 2010 and Lilly of the valley was presented to the Princess by Harold`s Great Great Granddaughter, Mia Pearlman. The value of the medals was such that each year we have been able to endow a medical scholarship which runs for a duration of four years and there is an annual medical lecture. Sixteen scholars have now been elected, eleven of whom have now qualified. This is a brief history of Harold's life, Doctor, Scientist & Gentleman.

"At the going down of the sun and in the morning we will remember them."

Mia Pearlman presents Lillies of the Valley to the Princess Royal

Dr Eubulus Williams and the Bristol Children's Hospital

DR MICHAEL WHITFIELD
Presented to the Bristol Medico-Historical Society June 2015

As we are meeting this evening in Henleaze, the story starts appropriately with one of the Ormerod doctors. The Ormerods had been doctors in Bristol continuously from the late 18th century until I arrived in Bristol in the 1960s. The last Ormerod practised from the surgery on the corner of Henleaze Road and Westbury Road – the house is now a residential home for the elderly.

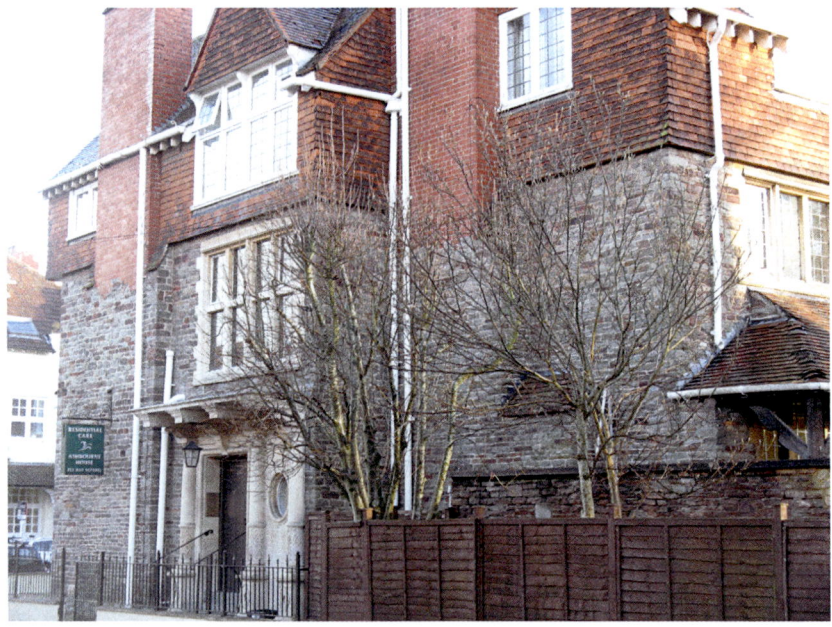

Henry Ormerod was the Ormerod doctor involved in the start of the Children's Hospital. He was one of the sons of the surgeon William Ormerod and was born in 1834 in Portland Square in the centre of Bristol.

In 1857 one of Henry Ormerod's brothers-in-law, Mortimer Granville who was either the partner of his father or his elder brother, opened a private dispensary for women and children at 17 Lower Castle St and Henry became associated with it. In 1858 the Institution moved to a house in St James Square where it became known as The Free Institution for the treatment of diseases peculiar to Women and Children. Henry Ormerod and Mortimer Granville took it in turns to be duty doctor to the Institution for a week at a time. Attendances of patients were about ten women and between thirty and forty children a week.

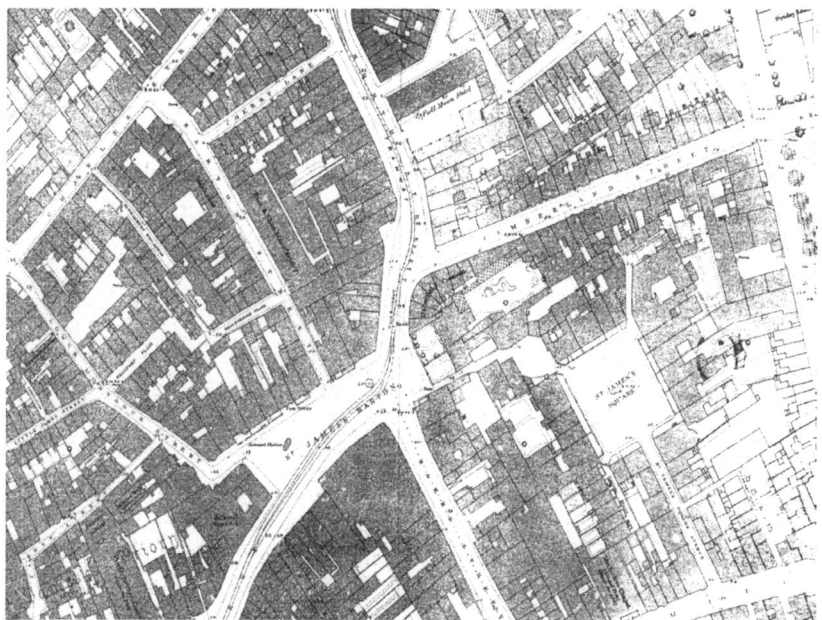

Map of Bristol 1911 showing St James' Square to the right of St James Barton

Mortimer Granville left his wife and family and moved to London shortly after 1861 where he lived with his sister and followed a successful career as a physician and medical journalist writing for *The Lancet*. In 1877 he produced a two volume book called the *Care and Cure of the Insane* following *The Lancet's* investigation of the London asylums. His great claim to fame though was his invention of his electrical percuteur which produced rapid vibrations to be applied to the skin to reduce a patient's pain such as in Trigeminal neuralgia and headaches. Originally called a percusser or more colloquially *"Granville's hammer"*, the machine was manufactured and sold to physicians, but as it became increasingly popular its inventor tried to disassociate himself from the device's *"mis-use"*. In his 1883 book on the subject, *Nerve-Vibration and Excitation as Agents in the Treatment of Functional Disorder and Organic Disease*, he wrote, *"I have never yet percussed a female patient ... I have avoided, and shall continue to avoid the treatment of women by percussion, simply because I do not wish to be hoodwinked, and help to mislead others, by the vagaries of the hysterical state ..."*

Nevertheless in 2011 a romantic comedy was produced called *Hysteria* that described how Dr Mortimer Granville produced his vibrator to help in the treatment of Hysteria.

In 1858 at the first annual meeting of the Free Institution, *Eubulus Williams* was appointed assistant medical officer.

He continued as a surgeon to the Institution until 1862 when he resigned as a result of pressure from his private practice[1] but, as he later

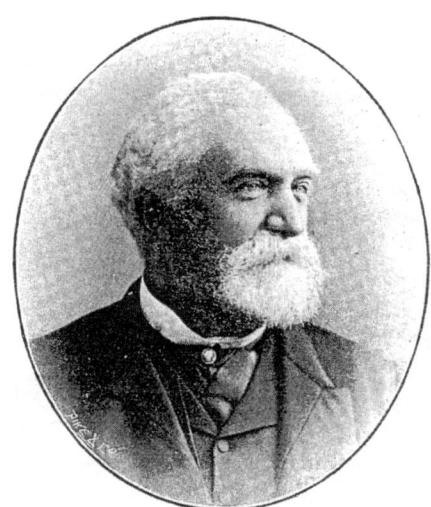

Dr. Eubulus Williams.

claimed, at the repeated requests of one of the staff he resumed his job.

Eubulus Williams was born in Williton, Somerset on July 20th 1831. He was educated at Taunton College. Like three of his brothers he trained at Guys Hospital in London. He then worked for a year as a house surgeon in the Reading Hospital and then spent three years as the medical superintendent at the Dundee Royal Infirmary from 1855. He obtained his MD at St Andrews in 1855. His obituary[2] stated that *'He afterwards visited the medical schools in Berlin, Paris and Vienna to study their different modes of treatment, attending lectures and receiving certificates from the various professors.'*

According to his granddaughter, he had made a run-away match with the beautiful Miss Watson whom he married in 1858. He commenced practice in Bristol in that year following the example of his elder doctor brother Joseph who had died during Bristol's second cholera epidemic ten years earlier (1849). In 1864 he advertised in the Bristol Mercury stating: *'To the Committee and Subscribers of the Bristol Royal Infirmary. I have the honour to inform you that at the next vacancy in the Surgical Staff of your Infirmary I shall offer myself as a candidate. From the numerous offers of support that have been promised I am encouraged to hope that I shall, by your favours, be successful.'*

During the next few years several other doctors started working for the Free Institution in St James Square: Dr Henderson as Honorary Physician, and the surgeons Carter, Baretti, McDonald and Steele.

Dr Henderson (b 1825) who held the MRCP and MD, married Hester in 1853 and they lived in Richmond Hill, Clifton and had three children. However, the marriage ended in an acrimonious divorce after Henderson left for America with another woman in 1863.

Thomas Baretti (b 1834 in Bath) lived in Royal York Crescent. He replaced Henry Ormerod and went on to become a surgeon at the Clifton Dispensary and lived in Royal York Crescent; William Grover Carter was born in Guernsey in 1817 and lived in Bellevue, Clifton, held the MRCP and in 1863 he resigned as a surgeon to the Institution and was appointed physician. He had a very long association with the children's hospital becoming secretary in 1866.

James McDonald b 1821 was appointed in 1863 and died in 1866 and had his practice in High Kingsdown.

Charles Steele[3] qualified in 1860; obtained the FRCS in 1869 and his MD in1880. He was born at Macclesfield, where his father, the Rev John Steele, held the living of Christ Church, and he studied at the Bristol Medical School. He was elected Surgeon to the Free Institution in 1864 and District Medical Officer for Clifton. He became Surgeon to the Royal Infirmary in 1870, and lectured on physiology in the Medical School. He was for a time Secretary, and then Member of Council, of the Bath and Bristol Branch of the British Medical Association. He built up a large practice, both general and as a consultant, retiring from the Infirmary about 1908. He died in 1914.

The next key date in the history of the Children's Hospital was 1864, soon after *Mr Mark Whitwill* visited Great Ormond St Hospital and decided to start a similar institution in Bristol. Whitwill was a Yorkshire man who was born in Scarborough in 1827. He was a wealthy shipbroker who lived in one of the large houses that were later combined to form the Hawthorns Hotel – now part of the University. In 1863 his second son died at the age of three, so it was not surprising that he was primed to get involved in founding a children's hospital. Whitwill received an invitation from the St James Square dispensary to join their committee and realised that converting the dispensary into a hospital was a practical idea and the Bristol Children's Hospital opened in 1866. Fundraising occurred in 1865 and Whitwill became treasurer.

At the special general meeting of subscribers and donors, held in the new hospital on August 25th 1866, Mark Whitwill was the chairman and Dr Carter was the Hon. Secretary. The chairman said that the new premises had plenty of fresh air and light; it was a house adapted for the purpose of an infant institution and there was a nice piece of land attached to it. There would be no noise and £300 was needed to pay for the premises. The house was number 9 at the Royal Fort on the left hand side at the top of Royal Fort Road. The first patient was admitted on 26th October and there was only one room with nine cots. In December1867 there were nineteen children inpatients and during the previous week seventy-six women had been seen in outpatients and one hundred and thirty-one children.

It became the *Bristol Hospital for Sick Children and for the Outdoor Treatment of Women* and its objects were:
1. To provide for the reception, maintenance and medical and surgical treatment of the children of the poor under ten years during sickness in a light and airy building, salubriously placed; to furnish with advice and medicine those who cannot or need not be admitted into the hospital. And also to receive as outpatients women suffering from diseases peculiar to their sex.
2. To promote the advancement of medical science with reference to the diseases of women and children and especially to provide for the instruction of students in these essential departments of medical knowledge.
3. To diffuse among all classes of the community and particularly among the poor, a better acquaintance with the management of infants and children during health and sickness, and to assist in the education and training of women in the special duties of Christian nurses.

Expansion took place quickly – by 1868 there were four wards with twenty-four beds; next year a bronchial ward was added making thirty beds and in 1871 there were forty beds. In 1873 there was an infectious

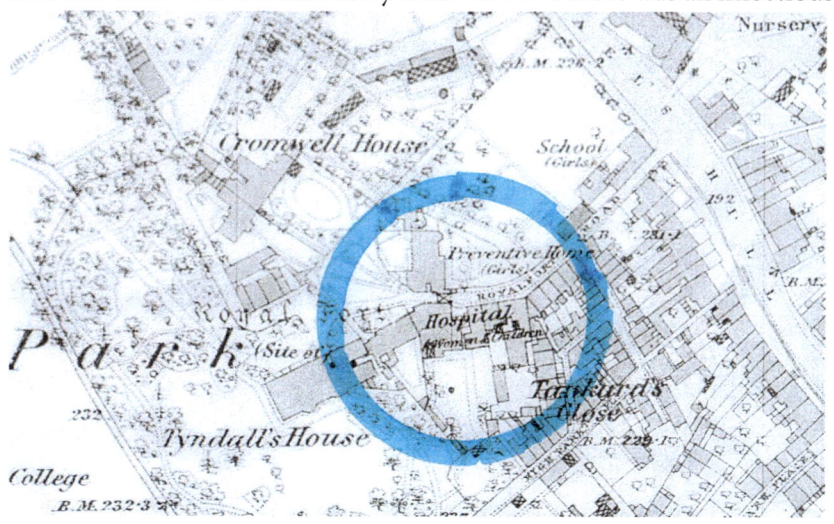

Map of 1885 indicating the site of the new hospital (now replaced by the Medical School building in Royal Fort Road)

ward added and in 1876 a room was added for women needing an operation, who were expected to pay 8 shillings a week. The present large site was bought in 1881.

We now return to Eubulus Williams who resigned his position as surgeon to the Childrens' Hospital in April 1867 when the rest of the staff threatened to resign in a body if he did not do so. Williams had published a document describing his conversion to Homoeopathy, a very brave or foolish thing to do as the 1850s and 60s were a time when there was much antagonism to homoeopathy. The fact that one of the other surgeons, Charles Steele was involved in the council of the local branch of the BMA would have made William's position particularly difficult. Williams' statement of conversion to homoeopathy that he sent to the Committee and Subscribers of the Bristol Hospital for Sick Children was published and in the British Journal of Homoeopathy it's reviewer stated:[4]

'Dr Williams is the most recent convert of Homoeopathy from among the ranks of our brethren of the old school. Holding, as he does, and has done for nine years past, the office of surgeon to a public institution, he feels it due to the Committee and Subscribers to announce his change of views, leaving it with them to decide whether they still desire to retain his services. We hope that those to whom it is addressed ... will not dismiss an old and tried servant because he has modified his treatment. For ourselves, we heartily welcome Dr Williams to our little band.'

The committee had no choice but to accept his resignation. In the local newspaper there was some correspondence between Williams and someone signing himself *'audi alteram partem'* (meaning from another point of view). From the contents of the letters the author was almost certainly Steele and the readers of the correspondence must have been surprised that two doctors were prepared to write to each other over this public spat.

Following his resignation Williams was appointed medical officer to the Muller's Orphanage, a position he held for thirty-four years. It was reported that he rode in the first carriage of Revd George Muller's funeral procession in 1898, an indication of the close relationship he held with that great man.

Eubulus Williams and his wife were active in the civic life of Bristol.

For instance in 1874 he was, as far as I can see, the only doctor present at a public meeting in the Colston Hall against the *Contagious Diseases Acts* that came into being between 1860 and 1880[5] in an attempt to control venereal diseases.

A special meeting of the *Bristol and Clifton Anti Vivisection Society* was held at their house in Lansdown Place on May 21 1883[6] and Williams was present at a meeting of the Governors of Clifton College on March 26th 1896 [7] but was never a member of College council.

He was President of the *West of England Therapeutical Society* from its formation until 1903. and in 1898 was President of the *British Homoeopathic Congress*. The subject of his Presidential Address at the Homoeopathic Congress was medical progress and he illustrated his talk with examples of physicians who had gone against contemporary wisdom. He mentioned Jenner about whom he wrote *'the profession shook its head when in 1798, after 25 years of patient investigations in the meadows of his native valleys, he came to London full of his discovery of the potency of cow-pox inoculation to give immunity of man from smallpox, the terrible scourge of that time, which annually claimed some 40,000 victims'* and he said *'failed to enlist the sympathy or help of his professional brethren, and after three months of ineffectual work (in London) he retired again to the country, there to prepare and in the same year to publish his treatise.'*

He then went on to talk about Samuel Hahnemann who introduced homoeopathy as a similar medical pioneer and said that *'his life and work are too recent and revolutionary to have won the world's praise as yet... and that it is encouraging to remember that the heterodoxy of one age frequently becomes the orthodoxy of the next'.*[8]

I have only found one example of a published article by Williams, that of a paper that was read originally to the Western Counties Therapeutic Society on *'The Medicinal Treatment of Nasal Polypi'.*[9] It is quite a short paper and the introduction gives a good indication of Williams' attitudes:

'To suggest remedial treatment (of nasal polyps) by medicine appears absurd in the face of the advocates of surgical removal of polypi, by the aid of electric cautery or snare.

I suppose we do not forget the able paper read by Dr Alexander on this disease; how enthusiastically he advocated the use of the electric snare, until one was almost tempted to wish one had a polypus for the pleasure of demonstrating in person the pleasantness of the operation. Indeed, so far did this prevail, that one of our number submitted to the position of "the operated". On the other hand there exist many exceptions to those who like to submit themselves to operation, and it is to encourage these timid ones that I bring forward some cases to illustrate the advantage of medication in the removal of these polypi.

While the electric snare is so great an improvement on the orthodox treatment of my early days, that by torsion, I should myself prefer medication. At the same time I would not oppose the operation to those who like it. If the cases I lay before should evoke sufficient interest to try the medicinal treatment, my object will be gained; as, if successful, they will be rewarded by the gratitude of a patient – and if unsuccessful, the operation can always be fallen back upon if necessary.'

He then described one case:

'*She visited me weekly for 6 weeks. I gave from the beginning merc. iod. 3x, three or four times daily. On her last visit her report was, in her own language, "I am all right now, it came away like a spring snail".*

Williams died on 9th January 1905 aged 74 after a long period of poor health and his Times obituary [10], probably written by his eldest son *Patrick Watson Williams* who became the Bristol's first ENT surgeon, stated that '*he was one of the most broad-minded and philanthropic of*

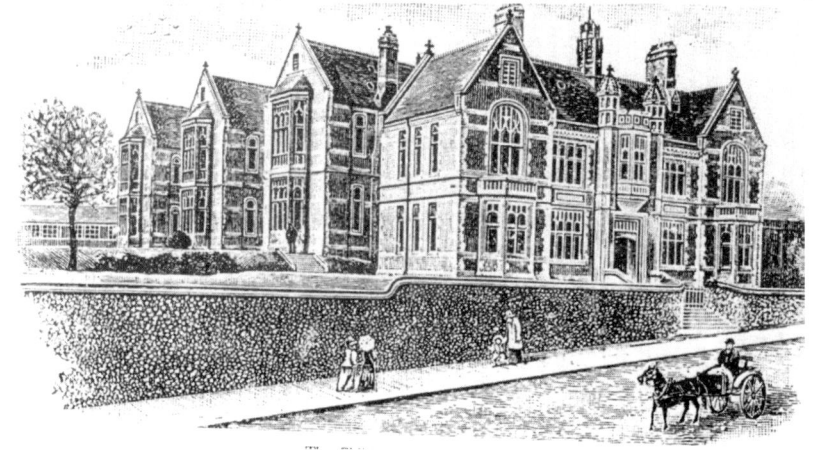

men'. He was described as a striking figure, tall, handsome, dignified, and distinctly distinguished looking – one that any passing stranger would remark and feel inclined to ask who he was. He was genial and kindly in manner, devoted to his profession, and much esteemed and loved by all who knew him, both patients and friends, to whom his departure will make a sad blank. He was much interested in religious and philanthropic movements, and always exerted his influence in the right direction.

References

1. Bristol Times and Daily Post 10 April 1867
2. Obituary The Times 17 Jan 1905
3. Plarr's Lives of surgeons at http://livesonline.rcseng.ac.uk/
4. British Journal of Homoeopathy 1867 Vol XXV p 473
5. Bristol Mercury Oct 17 1874
6. Bristol Mercury May 21 1883
7. Bristol Mercury March 26th 1896
8. Monthly Homoeopathic Review July 1 1898 p398
9. Monthly Homoeopathic Review Aug 1 1895 p426
10. Obituary The Times 17 Jan 1905

This paper was erroneously omitted from Volume VII of the Proceedings.

Tuberculous Meningitis (TBM)
ROY CRABBE AND JOHN POWELL
December 2012

This paper by Roy Crabbe formed the basis of a poster and handout prepared by John Powell and displayed at the Bristol Medico-Historical Society meeting.

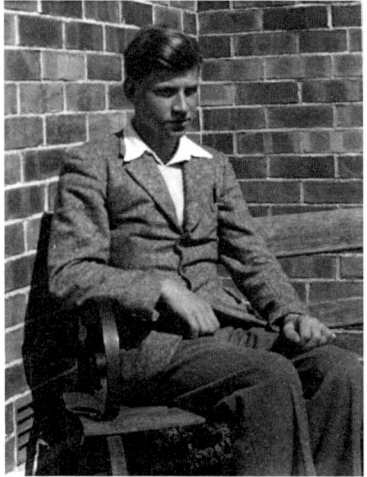
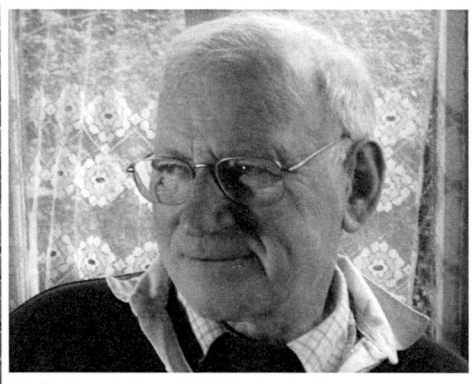

Left: Roy behind T block 1952
Above: Roy in 2012

My involvement with Ham Green really starts in July of 1951 after my mother had been diagnosed with Pulmonary TB after two years of treatment for chronic bronchitis (!) and two months after my sixteenth birthday. For several months I had not been too well myself and in the beginning of August I was admitted to the Lyme Regis Cottage hospital with pulmonary TB.

Not being in a fever hospital, I was quickly removed from Lyme to North Allington Isolation Hospital, Bridport, Dorset. At this time, and Ham Green hospital was one, most ports around the country had an isolation hospital providing some way of isolating those who entered the country by sea with contagious diseases. North Allington was the one for West Dorset. Gradually many of these hospitals were closed or became TB sanatoria.

About two weeks before my admission to this hospital on 21st August 1951, another very ill man, Eric Sykes, from Bridport, had been a patient with TB. He had become desperately ill, diagnosed with TB meningitis (TBM) and sent to Ham Green.

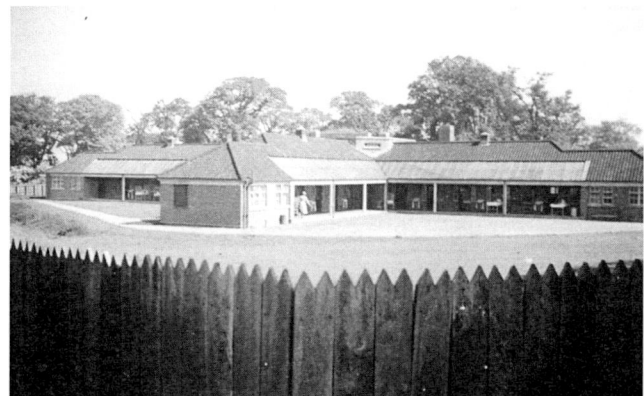

T block with its isolation fence

Although I do not remember feeling particularly ill at that time I guess that I must have been as I did not wish to get out of bed and presented other symptoms to the medical staff. After two days I was approached by the Ward Sister who told me that she suspected that I had TBM but that the visiting doctor disagreed. Of course, after Eric's recent sojourn the nursing staff were very aware of TBM which was killing most of the sufferers at this time. I remember a showdown between the Sister and the reluctant doctor where she said that if he would not take a CSF sample by Lumbar Puncture (LP) she would do it herself. The doctor gave in and the result is history. I was packed off to Ham Green the next day to join Eric in T ward.

I did not see Eric until the next Spring as he was in a single side room to himself and I was in a seven-bed ward: all of us with TBM. I think Eric was so ill that he needed special nursing. Eric eventually was able to get out of bed but, very sadly, died about July/August 1952: he had been married for only a couple of months before his illness.

The treatment was an initial eight weeks of intrathecal streptomycin daily (i.e., via LP into the subarachnoid space in the spine) and then very careful monitoring against a relapse. Most male patients that I saw made an initial recovery but died after a relapse. I was the first male TBM patient to be discharged, cured from TBM at Ham Green for over a year although there was a steady stream of patients. Many of these I did not see, as they died soon after arrival in single bedrooms, adjacent to the main ward.

There were more surviving female patients. Two girls, Heather

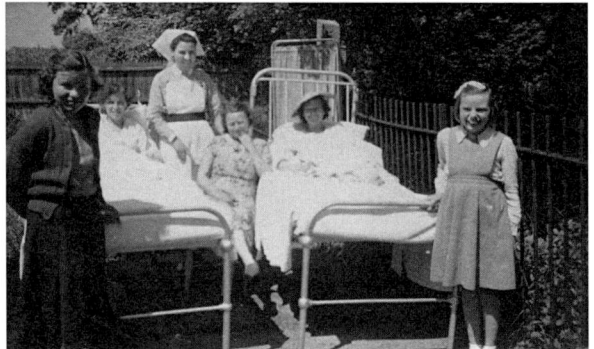

Standing left: Heather, Sister Canning and Christine

Brown and Christine, and an elder woman were discharged in my time: August 1951 – June 1952.

Lumbar punctures day after day for eight weeks were quite painful. OK to start with but the injection sites, limited to the lumbar region L3/L4, L4/L5, became inflamed and sore and the nerve running down the spine was often touched by the needle giving a dreadful sciatica-like pain running down your leg. If unsuccessful, the streptomycin had to be inserted via a cisternal puncture in the back of the neck. The neck was shaved and the injection pretty painless. As the needle would be very close to the brain, the doctors were reluctant to use this pathway very often.

At first, one would dread the clanking arrival of the LP trolley, nurse and doctor but in the end we would not hear it as we were, mostly, deafened by the streptomycin. At the bottom of my bed was a little boy in a cot about 18 months old and as soon as he heard the trolley he would scream and scream: he knew what was coming. We would lie on our side while the nurse would lean over the bed, enfold us behind the knees and neck and bend our spines as much as possible to open the vertebrae a bit and make it easier for the doctor and also to stop us jumping all over the bed when the needle hit the nerve. Most LPs were performed by a Dr McKendrick but just occasionally when he was away or when he could not get in, Dr Macrae the hospital superintendent would take the rounds. Dr James Macrae was a brilliant technician. First of all he had a special needle which was already attached to the syringe containing the streptomycin. He would just rub his finger along your spine, insert the needle painlessly and inject – marvellous. Sister

Williams was brilliant at holding us. Although a rather strict type, she was the epitome of the nursing profession. Later she was replaced by Sister Canning – I think Irish but a much friendlier type.

I digress to describe the nursing we received in Ward T. This was of the highest standard. I did not leave my bed once for eight months and, although I never wet the bed, there was always a red rubber sheet just under the cotton sheet one was lying on. This was perfect for producing bed sores but the many and regular back rubs we had prevented any of these. We were waited on, fed, bottled, bedpanned, wiped and bed bathed without fail or delay. A red letter day which has stuck clearly in my memory was when I first staggered to the toilet after about nine months of bedpans.

Since I left Ham Green I have met quite a few survivors of TBM. The staff at Ham Green with regard to treating relapsed cases, I think, could have been more vigorous in giving last ditch treatment which might have saved some. I may be very wrong about this but that is the impression I gained after meeting patients from other hospitals several of whom had had two or even three courses of streptomycin and recovered even after losing consciousness for days between sessions.

Visitors had to wear long capes or gowns if they went into wards and visiting times were limited. When we became ambulant we were able to walk around the hospital, meet patients with different diseases and even go for trips outside.

Below: The Avon estuary before the Avon Bridge was constructed

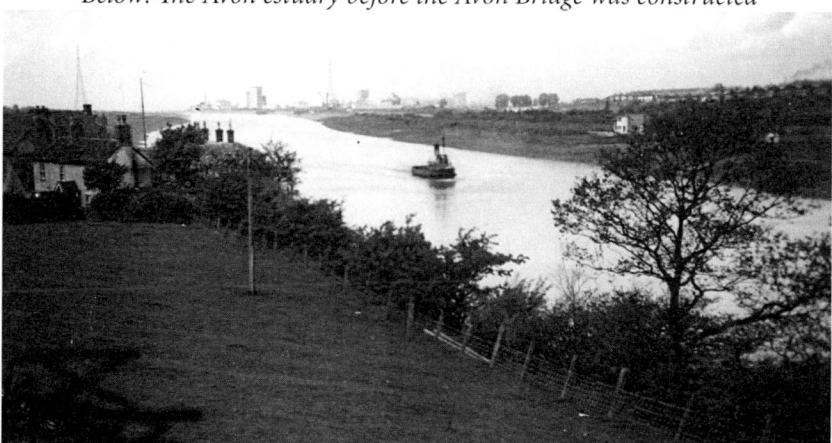

Very few patients recovered unscathed from TBM. Most of us were deafened to some extent and many, like myself, totally so. Normally this would have been very concerning and worrying for a patient but not so on our ward. The thing was TO SURVIVE first and be very happy if you did. After forty-five years I have regained a lot of hearing due to Cochlear Implants; a great bonus.

Meningitis also often scars the surface of the brain and causes epilepsy thereafter. This happened to me and, although then I went for fifty-one years without a seizure, unfortunately, the epilepsy has returned to haunt me.

In my time there, small boats plied the Avon Estuary and this was before the building of the bridge. Unfortunately, I did not explore Ham Green itself or up the riverside although we did wander over some of the fields around the hospital. Others have documented the history and fate of the hospital[1-4]: it will remain in my memory forever.

Roy Crabbe 2012

References and Notes

1. In 1899 Ham Green Hospital (76 beds) was opened as an isolation hospital, mainly to take care of typhoid cases. Over the next half century it developed into a large fever hospital (360 beds) and a sanatorium for patients with pulmonary tuberculosis (200 beds). In the 1950s it pioneered mechanical ventilation in respiratory failure during the poliomyelitis epidemics and opened the first intensive care unit in Bristol, eight years before the Bristol Royal Infirmary. In the 1960s it led the development of haemodialysis for acute renal failure in the SW region. Demand for infectious diseases beds fell in the 60s/70s and thereafter. The hospital was closed in 1997. See also:
2. Gerald Hart 1990. Ham Green. Crewkerne Books, Bristol. IBSN 0 9516074 0 5
3. John Powell 2006. Poliomyelitis in Bristol. Proc Brist Med-Hist Soc lV:175, abridged from www.johnpowell.net/pages/clevedon.htm
4. John Powell 2009. Bugs and Ham Green, Proc Brist Med-Hist Soc 2009; Va:102, abridged from www.johnpowell.net/pages/macrae.htm.

This paper was erroneously omitted from Volume VII of the Proceedings

In memorium:

On Monday 9 December 2019 Trevor Thomas gave a very interesting talk entitled *El Greco through Medical Eyes*. The evening was enjoyed by all. Sadly Trevor Thomas died at the beginning of August 2020.

Also in memorium
Tony Dickens and Chris Burns-Cox both died in 2018.

All sadly missed.

The Bristol Medico-Historical Society

Programme 2016-2020

19 September 2016 (AGM)
Dr Nabil Jarad: A history of the management of Emphysema
Dr Peter Carpenter: Two madhouses of St Georges

12 December 2016
Prof Brian Vincent: Two medical chemists of Bristol - Beddoes and Herepath.

24 April 2017
Prof T F Baskett: A History of Caesarian Birth.

Monday 16th October 2017 (AGM)
Janet Sellick: Agatha Christie's use of poison in her novels.

Monday 11th December 2017
Prof Peter Dunn: Sir Francis Bacon [1561-1626], philosopher, polymath, poet and playwright.

Monday 19th March 2018
Dr Jonathan Musgrave: An introduction to Leonardo Da Vinci's anatomical drawings
Dr M Whitfield: Dr Richard Smith

30 April 2018
Prof T F Baskett: Frank Pantridge and the Evolution of Pre-hospital Emergency Care
Dr Roger Rolls: the Bath Medical History Museum.

15 October 2018 (AGM)
Dr P Mains: the Hotwells Spa
Judith Franklin: the later life of Elizabeth Dunbar.

10 December 2018
Lois M Tutton – All I want to Christmas is my two front teeth.
Prof Paul Goddard - History of MRI

Monday 11 March 2019
Prof Peter Dunn – Swaddling: then and now
Prof Gordon Stirrat: The Poppy: panacea and plague

Monday 3 June 2019
Dr Bruno Bubna-Kasteliz: Scottish doctors at the Russian Imperial Court
Dr Mike Davidson – Scottish doctors and the slave trade

Monday 14 October 2019 (AGM)
Mr Walford Gillison: Vesalius, the angry father of human anatomy
Prof Francis Duck Bath War Hospital (1916-1919)

Monday 9 December 2019
Dr Trevor Thomas: El Greco through Medical Eyes

March 9 2020
Prof Peter Dunn: John Dunn and the Zulu War
Mr. Chris Ackroyd: The history of the Victoria Cross